First Aid for Families
A Parent's Guide to Safe and Healthy Kids

American Academy of Pediatrics

DEDICATED TO THE HEALTH OF ALL CHILDREN™

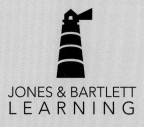

JONES & BARTLETT
LEARNING

American Academy of Pediatrics

DEDICATED TO THE HEALTH OF ALL CHILDREN™

World Headquarters
Jones & Bartlett Learning
40 Tall Pine Drive
Sudbury, MA 01776
978-443-5000
info@jblearning.com
www.jblearning.com

Jones & Bartlett Learning Canada
6339 Ormindale Way
Mississauga, Ontario L5V 1J2
Canada

Jones & Bartlett Learning International
Barb House, Barb Mews
London W6 7PA
United Kingdom

Adapted from *Pediatric First Aid for Caregivers and Teachers*
  by Brenda D. Schoolfield
Medical Editor: Susan Fuchs, MD, FAAP, FACEP
Managing Editor: Thaddeus Anderson, Manager, Life Support Programs
Marilyn Bull, MD, FAAP, AAP Board Reviewer
Robert Perelman, MD, FAAP, Director, Department of Education
Wendy Simon, MA, CAE, Director, Life Support Programs
Rebecca Bretaña, Life Support Assistant

American Academy of Pediatrics
141 Northwest Point Boulevard
Post Office Box 927
Elk Grove Village, IL 60009-0927
847-434-4000
www.aap.org

Jones & Bartlett Learning books and products are available through most bookstores and online booksellers. To contact Jones & Bartlett Learning directly, call 800-832-0034, fax 978-443-8000, or visit our website, www.jblearning.com.

Substantial discounts on bulk quantities of Jones & Bartlett Learning publications are available to corporations, professional associations, and other qualified organizations. For details and specific discount information, contact the special sales department at Jones & Bartlett Learning via the above contact information or send an email to specialsales@jblearning.com.

Production Credits
Chairman, Board of Directors: Clayton Jones
Chief Executive Officer: Ty Field
President: James Homer
Sr. V.P., Chief Operating Officer: Don W. Jones, Jr.
V.P., Design and Production: Anne Spencer
V.P., Manufacturing and Inventory Control: Therese Connell
Executive Publisher: Kimberly Brophy
Executive Acquisitions Editor—EMS: Christine Emerton
Associate Production Editor: Lisa Cerrone

Marketing Manager: Brian Rooney
Composition: Spoke & Wheel
Cover Design: Anne Spencer
Associate Photo Researcher: Jessica Elias
Cover and Title Page Images: Clockwise from top:
  © Monkey Business Images/ShutterStock, Inc.;
  © Monkey Business Images/ShutterStock, Inc.;
  © get4net/ShutterStock, Inc.
Printing and Binding: Courier Kendallville
Cover Printing: Courier Stoughton

The procedures and protocols in this book are based on the most current recommendations of responsible medical sources. The American Academy of Pediatrics and the publisher, however, make no guarantee as to, and assume no responsibility for, the correctness, sufficiency, or completeness of such information or recommendations. Other or additional safety measures may be required under particular circumstances.

This textbook is intended solely as a guide to the appropriate procedures to be employed when rendering emergency care to the sick and injured. It is not intended as a statement of the standards of care required in any particular situation, because circumstances and the patient's physical condition can vary widely from one emergency to another. Nor is it intended that this textbook shall in any way advise emergency personnel concerning legal authority to perform the activities or procedures discussed. Such local determination should be made only with the aid of legal counsel.

Additional illustration and photographic credits appear on page 236, which constitutes a continuation of the copyright page.

Library of Congress Cataloging-in-Publication Data
First aid for families : a parent's guide to safe and healthy kids / American Academy of Pediatrics.
    p. cm.
  ISBN 978-0-7637-5552-2 (pbk.)
  1. Pediatric emergencies. 2. First aid in illness and injury.
  RJ370.F583 2010
  618.92'0025—dc22
                                                                      2010040553

6048
Printed in the United States of America
15 14 13 12 11   10 9 8 7 6 5 4 3 2 1

American Academy of Pediatrics
DEDICATED TO THE HEALTH OF ALL CHILDREN™

Dear Parents and Families:

As a parent, keeping our children healthy and safe is our number one priority. But, from time to time, accidents happen. Whether it is a scrape on the knee or something more serious like choking on a piece of food, it is imperative for parents and caregivers to be prepared to provide first aid to their children. Learning first aid skills is an important step in ensuring a healthy environment for your loved ones.

First Aid for Families: A Parent's Guide to Safe and Healthy Kids is a tremendous resource that gives parents the information to provide immediate care to an injured child. You will find useful information such as The Six Steps of Pediatric First Aid, and helpful sections like "What You Should Look For" and "What You Should Do" on specific first aid topics. Additionally, one chapter provides you valuable information on how to address more complicated emergencies such as breathing problems, cardiopulmonary resuscitation (CPR), and choking relief for infants, children, and adolescents.

Utilizing your child's pediatrician, this book, and our parent-focused website, Healthy Children (www.healthychildren.org), will provide you with the information and tools needed to ensure a safe and healthy lifestyle for your family.

Thank you for your commitment to your child's well-being.

Sincerely,

Errol R. Alden, MD, FAAP
Executive Director/CEO
American Academy of Pediatrics

CONTENTS

What Is Pediatric First Aid?

What Is Pediatric First Aid?

Pediatric first aid is medical care that you give right away to a child who is injured or suddenly becomes very sick (**Figure 1**). Parents and caregivers need to know what to do for minor injuries as well as for emergency situations. **Caregivers** can include legal

pediatric first aid The medical care that you give right away to a child who is injured or suddenly becomes very sick.

caregivers Legal guardians, relatives, and others who care for children.

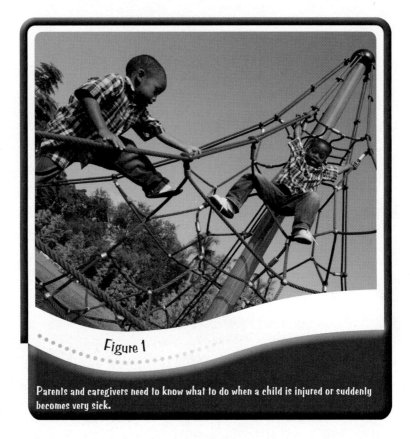

Parents and caregivers need to know what to do when a child is injured or suddenly becomes very sick.

guardians, relatives, and others who care for children. Most injuries that require first aid are not life-threatening emergencies. Usually first aid involves simple, commonsense procedures. However, first aid can sometimes mean the difference between life and death.

CPR An abbreviation for cardiopulmonary resuscitation; CPR is emergency first aid for someone who is not responding and not breathing. To give CPR, the rescuer alternates compressing the chest to help keep blood circulating and giving rescue breaths to get air into the child's lungs. If available, an AED (automated external defibrillator) is used to help the heart start beating again.

All parents and caregivers should have pediatric first aid training (**Figure 2**). This book is designed to help you handle many types of childhood medical situations. You will learn what to look for to decide if your child needs emergency care. Many people use the term cardiopulmonary resuscitation or **CPR** to refer to all first aid skills. This is not correct. CPR focuses on what to do when the heart stops beating or when a child cannot breathe. It doesn't include what to do for other types of situations where your child might need first aid. For example, it doesn't teach you what to do when a child falls and scrapes his knee.

Children do not often need CPR. If a child is healthy, his heart usually keeps beating unless he stops breathing. Some reasons that breathing might stop are choking, drowning, or a rare heart condition. When breathing stops, the heart will eventually quit beating. For this reason, all parents and caregivers need to know what to do if a child is choking. You also need to know how to give rescue breaths. **Rescue breathing** is a way to get air back into the lungs of a child who is not breathing.

rescue breathing A technique for getting air back into the lungs of a child who is not breathing.

This book contains first aid steps for choking. It also contains steps for rescue breathing and CPR. You may want to consider taking a community class in CPR for parents and caregivers. A class will give you a chance to practice CPR and improve your skills. CPR video kits are available for learning these important skills at home.

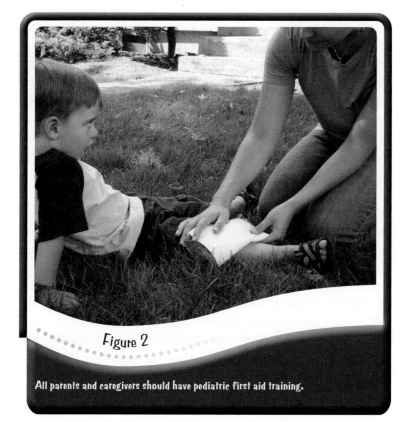

Figure 2

All parents and caregivers should have pediatric first aid training.

3

Parents often have other people's children in their care. If any child in your care becomes injured or suddenly very sick, you should not hesitate to give first aid. Most states have a **Good Samaritan Law** that protects someone who gives first aid from lawsuits. Although laws vary from state to state, the Good Samaritan Law applies to a person who is trying to help in an emergency and is acting in good faith. The law protects the person from legal responsibility if she does what a reasonable person with the same amount of training would have done.

Good Samaritan Law A law passed in many states to protect someone from legal liability when giving first aid in an emergency.

How Will I Learn Pediatric First Aid?

The best way to learn pediatric first aid is to set aside some time to read this book. This book discusses many childhood illnesses and injuries that require first aid. You can use this book before, during, and after a medical situation:

Before: Read and study the entire book to learn important concepts. This will help you prepare for medical situations. Talk to your medical provider if you have questions about a particular topic.

During: Refer to specific chapters when your child is sick or injured to help figure out what is wrong. Look up the first aid care that your child needs. Use it to guide you in the best actions to take.

After: Read through information about the illness or injury again. Look for ways to keep your child safe. Take steps to prevent the problem from happening again, if possible.

Take a few minutes now and look through the book to see how it is organized. There are 15 chapters and 2 appendices.

Chapter 1 introduces you to the book. Chapter 2 gives important information about the Six Steps of Pediatric First Aid. You will use these steps to effectively handle every medical situation. Chapters 3 through 14 each focus on a specific type of illness or injury. Chapter 15 discusses ways to keep your child safe and things you can do to prevent illness and injury.

The appendices are divided into two parts. Appendix A gives brief information on common childhood illnesses, such as sore throat. Appendix B lists first aid supplies that you might need.

Each of the 15 chapters is divided into the following sections:

Introduction: an overview of the chapter.

What You Should Know: background information that gives you a basic understanding of the topic.

What You Should Look For: signs and symptoms that you should look for to help you figure out what is wrong with your child.

What You Should Do: a reminder to follow the Six Steps of Pediatric First Aid in every medical situation. These steps are followed by step-by-step instructions for first aid care.

You will see that key terms are in **bold type**. Definitions of these terms can be found in the margins and at the end of this book.

Each chapter also includes information in highlighted boxes. Some boxes give first aid tips or ways to keep your child safe. Other boxes review key points from the discussion or tell you where to get more information.

The Six Steps of Pediatric First Aid are included in each chapter. This is because you need to use these steps in every situation requiring first aid. These six steps are discussed in detail in Chapter 2. Be sure to take some time to read and study them. Following these steps will give you confidence. They will help you handle medical situations calmly and effectively.

The Six Steps of Pediatric First Aid

1 Evaluate the Situation

Take a few seconds to look around. Evaluate the situation. Make sure the surroundings are safe. Find out who is involved and what happened.

▼

2 Look and Listen for Signs of an Emergency

Look and listen for signs that your child's condition is serious or life threatening. Notice the ABCs (**A**ppearance, **B**reathing, and **C**irculation). Always call **emergency medical services (EMS)** for life-threatening conditions. To call EMS, dial 911.

emergency medical services (EMS) A system of trained medical professionals who handle out-of-hospital emergencies. EMS is linked to a nationwide emergency phone number. In the United States, dial 911 to contact EMS.

▼

Check for Problems

Take a closer look and check your child for problems. Use the "What You Should Look For" sections to guide you. Figure out what is wrong, how serious it is, and what you should do next.

▼

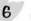 ### Act

Based on what is wrong, take action. Read the "What You Should Do" sections to be prepared. For a simple injury, you may only need to give first aid. For a serious condition, you may need to call EMS and give care until help arrives.

▼

Follow Up

Be sure to follow up. Give any care or treatment that your child might need after the event.

▼

Prevent

Take steps to prevent the illness or injury from happening again, if possible. Prevention is as important as first aid in caring for your child.

2

Six Steps of Pediatric First Aid

● Six Steps of Pediatric First Aid

Introduction

Your 8-year-old son falls off his bike and is lying in the street close to your driveway. Your 3-year-old daughter gets into the cleaning supplies in the bathroom and now is vomiting. Your 2-month-old baby has a fever of 103.6° F, and her breathing doesn't sound right. In each situation, you must take a calm, step-by-step approach to getting help and giving first aid.

What You Should Know

You need to be prepared to give first aid if your child gets hurt or becomes sick. Learn the Six Steps of Pediatric First Aid. This step-by-step approach will help you figure out what is wrong and what to do to provide the very best care for your child. Following these steps will help you stay calm and in control of any medical situation.

Six Steps of Pediatric First Aid

1 Evaluate the Situation

Take a few seconds to look around. Evaluate the situation. Make sure the surroundings are safe. Find out who is involved and what happened.

▼

2 Look and Listen for Signs of an Emergency

Look and listen for signs that your child's condition is serious or life threatening. Notice the ABCs (**A**ppearance, **B**reathing, and **C**irculation). Always call emergency medical services (EMS) for life-threatening conditions. To call EMS, dial 911.

▼

3 Check for Problems

Take a closer look and check your child for problems. Use the "What You Should Look For" sections to guide you. Figure out what is wrong, how serious it is, and what you should do next.

▼

4 Act

Based on what is wrong, take action. Read the "What You Should Do" sections to be prepared. For a simple injury, you may only need to give first aid. For a serious condition, you may need to call EMS and give care until help arrives.

▼

5 Follow Up

Be sure to follow up. Give any care or treatment that your child might need after the event.

▼

6 Prevent

Take steps to prevent the illness or injury from happening again, if possible. Prevention is as important as first aid in caring for your child.

What You Should Know

Step 1: Evaluate the Situation

As you approach a child who is sick or hurt, take a few seconds to look around. Evaluate the situation.

- Make sure the surroundings are safe.
- Find out who is involved.
- Find out what happened.

First, make sure that everyone there is safe, including you. Look for hazards, such as oncoming traffic, deep water, or fire. Other dangers are falling objects, a live electrical wire, or a dangerous animal. You may want to rush to your child right away, but don't ignore your own safety. You can't care for your child if you get hurt too.

It is best to comfort a child who is hurt without moving her. If the surroundings are not safe and you must move a child, take caution.

Be very careful moving anyone who may have fallen because a **spinal injury** *is possible.*

Do not move the child's head and neck. This could cause more damage to the spine. Use one of the methods described in **Table 1** to move a child based on the possibility of a spinal injury and the child's age.

Note: Encourage an injured child not to move if anything hurts. However, if a child can move without feeling pain, don't force her to hold still.

spinal injury An injury that damages the spinal cord; moving a child with a spinal injury incorrectly may cause more damage. Spinal injuries are very serious and can result in paralysis and death. If you must move a child with a suspected spinal injury to keep him safe, use the shoulder drag method.

Second, find out who is involved. Look for others who may be sick or hurt. A crying child may get your attention first, but others may be involved who have more serious conditions. Look for other children who may need to be kept from harm. Look for someone

Table 1 How to Move a Child

Spinal Injury Possible?	Method	Technique	Use for This Age
Yes	Shoulder drag (**Figure 1**)	• Place your hands under the child's shoulders. • Brace the child's neck by placing your forearms along the sides of the head. • Slowly drag the child to the nearest safe location, while continuing to brace the head and neck.	All ages
No	Cradle carry (**Figure 2A**)	Carry the child by cradling him in your arms.	Babies and younger children
No	Ankle drag (**Figure 2B**)	Slowly drag the child by his ankles.	Older children

who can watch them. See if there is another adult who can give first aid or call for help.

Third, find out what happened. Try to figure out what caused the illness or injury. If your child fell, try to find out the distance. You need to know if he fell off his bike or from the top of a tree. If he is bleeding, look for what could have caused it. He will need different care based on whether he cut himself on a rock, stepped on a rusty nail, or a stray animal bit him. Knowing the cause will help you make the best decisions about what to do next.

First Aid TIP

If you are not sure it is an emergency but are concerned, always call EMS. In most of the United States, you will dial 911. **If you are traveling or your community has a different EMS telephone number, be sure to find out the correct number to call** *before* **an emergency.**

What You Should Look For

Step 2: Look and Listen for Signs of an Emergency

Look and listen for signs that your child's condition is serious or life threatening before you do anything else. Many times you can tell if something is wrong with your child even if he is asleep. The purpose of this step is to decide if you should call EMS right

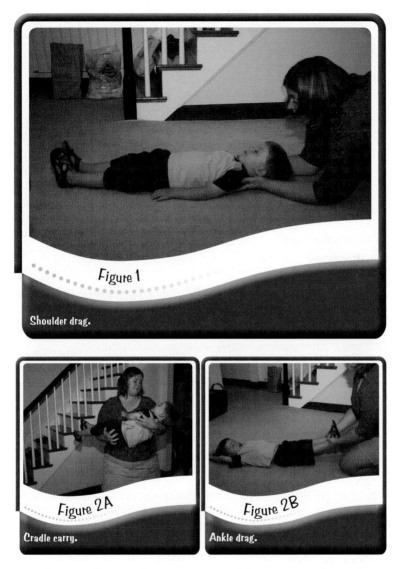

Figure 1

Shoulder drag.

Figure 2A

Cradle carry.

Figure 2B

Ankle drag.

away because the situation is urgent, or if the situation isn't urgent, but your child still needs to see a doctor for medical care. See **Table 2** for a list of conditions that are life-threatening emergencies when the best action is to call EMS. See **Table 3** for situations when your child needs medical care but doesn't need to be taken to a medical facility by an ambulance.

Use the ABCs (**A**ppearance, **B**reathing, **C**irculation) to guide you when looking and listening for signs that your child needs urgent medical care.

Table 2 When to Call EMS

Call Emergency Medical Services (EMS) immediately for the following:
- Any time you believe a child needs immediate medical treatment
- Fever in association with abnormal ABCs (appearance, breathing, or circulation)
- Multiple children affected by injury or serious illness at the same time
- A child is acting strangely, is much less alert, or is much more withdrawn
- Difficulty breathing, unable to speak
- Skin or lips that look blue, purple, or gray
- Rhythmic jerking of arms and legs and a loss of responsiveness (seizure)
- Unresponsive
- Decreasing responsiveness
- Any of the following after a head injury: decrease in level of alertness, confusion, headache, vomiting, irritability, difficulty walking
- Increasing or severe pain anywhere
- A cut or burn that is large and deep, and will not stop bleeding
- Vomiting blood
- A child with a severe stiff neck, headache, and fever
- A child who is significantly dehydrated: sunken eyes, not making tears or urinating, lethargic
- Suddenly spreading purple or red rash
- A large volume of blood in the stools
- Hot or cold weather injuries (e.g., frostbite, heat exhaustion)

Did You Know?

In many areas of the United States, EMS can identify the location of a 911 emergency call using special technology. Mobile phone calls, however, cannot always be identified. Always be prepared to tell the EMS dispatcher your exact location. At home keep your street address posted by the telephone.

Appearance: You can tell if your child is sick or hurt just by looking at him (**Table 4**). If your child's appearance is not normal, his condition may be life threatening. Always call EMS for life-threatening conditions.

Breathing: Breathing problems in a baby or child can be very serious (**Table 5**). See *Chapter 3: Breathing Problems* to learn more. Always call EMS if your child is having trouble breathing.

Circulation: If your child's skin color is not normal, there may be a problem (**Table 6**). Call EMS to assess

Table 3 Situations Requiring Medical Attention

Situations that do not necessarily require ambulance transport, but still need medical attention:

- Fever in any age child who looks more than mildly ill
- Fever of >100.5°F in a child younger than 60 days (2 months) old
- Any age child who appears and is acting very ill
- Severe vomiting and/or diarrhea
- A serious cut that may require stitches (i.e., a wound that does not hold together by itself after cleaning)
- Any animal bites that puncture the skin
- Any venomous bites or stings with spreading local redness and swelling, or evidence of general illness
- Any medical condition specifically outlined in a child's care plan requiring parental notification

Table 4 Appearance

	Normal Appearance	Not Normal Appearance
Alert	Opens eyes; makes eye contact; follows movement	Eyes are closed; opens eyes only if you speak to him; stares off at nothing
Responsive	Responds to your voice or to toys	Doesn't respond as usual or doesn't respond at all (unresponsive)
Moves	Moves arms and legs normally	Body is limp or stiff; arms and legs don't move

your child if the skin color is very pale (more than normal) or bluish (**Figure 3**). Call EMS if your child is bleeding and you can't get it to stop.

When babies are cold, you may notice a blotchy "marble-like" look to their skin. This is called **mottling**. Pale skin and mottling may be normal if the room temperature is cold. A baby's hands and feet may look bluish when cold. It is not normal for a

mottling A blotchy "marble-like" look to the skin.

Table 5 Breathing

	Normal Breathing	Having Trouble Breathing
Effort	Breathing is regular; child is not having trouble breathing	Child's nostrils flare as he breathes in; his abdomen or chest moves more than normal with each breath; child's head bobs up and down
Rate	Child seems to be breathing at a normal rate	Child is breathing faster than normal or has a strange breathing pattern
Breathing sounds	You can't hear any unusual sounds when the child breathes in and out	You hear wheezing, snoring, grunting, or gurgling noises with each breath. The child has a seal-like barking cough.
Position	Child is comfortable, both sitting up or lying down	Child is more comfortable in an upright position and doesn't want to lie down; he may be sitting upright and leaning forward taking very deep breaths
Voice or cry	Sounds normal	Child's voice is weak, hoarse, or muffled; he can only say a few words at a time
Anxiety	Does not seem anxious	Child is anxious or afraid because of trouble breathing

Table 6 Circulation

Sign	Normal	Not Normal
Skin color	Looks normal	• Very pale (more than normal) • Bluish • Blotchy or mottled • Very pink or red • Spreading purple or red rash
Bleeding	No bleeding	• Bleeding that won't stop • Bleeding under the skin

warm child to have these signs. A child whose skin is unusually pink may be overheated or have a rash. A spreading purple or red rash is a cause for concern.

What You Should Look For

Step 3: Check for Problems

Take a closer look and check your child for problems. Read through the "What You Should Look For" sections in this book to be prepared for many medical situations. Most of the time, your child's problem will be easy to handle. Minor childhood injuries can be taken care of with a few simple first aid steps. By knowing what you should look for in advance, you will be alert to signs and symptoms that are more serious.

What You Should Do

Step 4: Act

In every medical situation, follow the Six Steps of Pediatric First Aid. Stay calm and in control. Based on what is wrong, take action. Read through the "What You Should Do" sections in this book to be prepared to give first aid for many medical situations. For most medical situations, simple first aid steps will take care of the problem. Call your medical provider if you have questions or concerns. For life-threatening emergencies, always call EMS. Give first aid care until EMS providers arrive and take over.

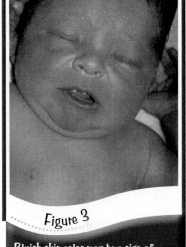

Figure 3

Bluish skin color may be a sign of a problem.

What You Should Do

Step 5: Follow Up

Follow-up care is just as important as first aid care. If your medical provider gives your child medicine, be sure that your child takes it as directed. Many times you will need to give the medicine until it is gone and not stop just because your child is feeling better. If your medical provider wants to see your child for a follow-up visit, make sure that happens.

Another important way to follow up is to be aware of things you can do to prevent illness or injury. See "Step 6: Prevent."

What You Should Do

Step 6: Prevent

Always be alert for things you can do to prevent illness or injury. Sometimes illnesses can be prevented by teaching your child and others in your family the importance of good hygiene. Simple things such as proper hand washing and coughing into the shoulder can reduce the spread of germs. You can prevent injury by making sure your home and your child's play areas are safe. An important example is prevention of choking. Choking can be a life-threatening emergency. You can take steps to prevent choking by being aware of possible choking hazards. Then identify any in your home and keep them away from your child. Another example is prevention of poisoning. You can keep your child safe by knowing what substances in your home are poisonous and making sure your child cannot get to them.

Ways to prevent illness and injury are discussed throughout this book. Prevention is as important as first aid in caring for your child. *Chapter 15: What Can I Do to Keep My Child Safe?* will help you recognize possible dangers. There are tips for keeping your child safe in specific rooms in your house, such as the kitchen and bathroom. There are other tips for keeping your child safe in and around cars, on bicycles, and around water. Encourage others who care for your child to use these tips to make sure their homes and play areas are safe.

Breathing Problems

Breathing Problems

Introduction

Breathing problems in a baby or child can be very serious. Always call EMS if your child is having trouble breathing or is not breathing. The body needs oxygen to live. The brain can survive for only a few minutes without oxygen (**Figure 1**). This is why it is an urgent,

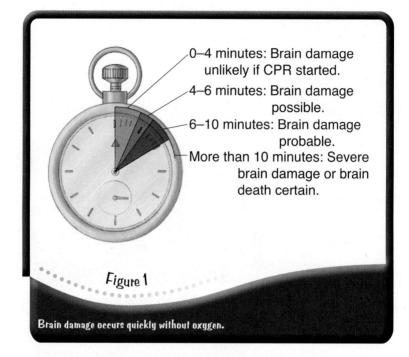

0–4 minutes: Brain damage unlikely if CPR started.

4–6 minutes: Brain damage possible.

6–10 minutes: Brain damage probable.

More than 10 minutes: Severe brain damage or brain death certain.

Figure 1

Brain damage occurs quickly without oxygen.

life-threatening emergency when a child stops breathing. All parents and caregivers should learn what to do if a child is choking. All parents and caregivers should learn how to do rescue breathing and CPR.

What You Should Know

The most common causes for breathing problems in babies and young children are respiratory infection, choking, and drowning. Asthma and allergic reactions may cause the airway to swell (**Figure 2**). This can cause breathing problems. When a child's heart stops beating, it is usually caused by the child's not being able to breathe. Brain damage can then occur within minutes. A child who is not breathing may die waiting for EMS to arrive unless you take quick action. Be sure to learn the first aid steps for a choking baby and child. Other important skills to learn are how to give rescue breathing and high-quality CPR.

Choking can be prevented. Food accounts for over 50% of choking episodes. Be alert for small objects that can

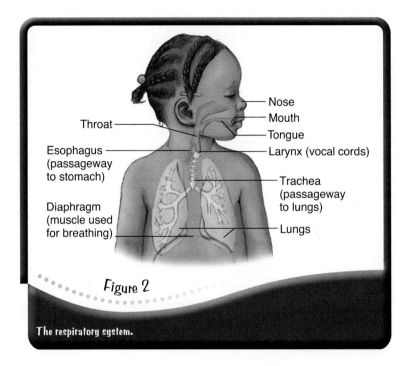

Throat

Esophagus (passageway to stomach)

Diaphragm (muscle used for breathing)

Nose

Mouth

Tongue

Larynx (vocal cords)

Trachea (passageway to lungs)

Lungs

Figure 2

The respiratory system.

cause choking, such as coins, buttons, and small toys. Check under furniture and between cushions for small items that children could find and put in their mouths. Toys are designed to be used by children within a certain age range. Age guidelines take into account the safety of a toy based on any possible choking hazard. Don't let young children play with toys designed for older children. Latex balloons are also a choking hazard. If a child bites a balloon and takes a breath, he could suck it into his airway.

Some foods can cause choking. Keep foods such as grapes, hot dogs, raw carrots, or peanuts away from babies and young children. Cut food for babies and young children into pieces no larger than one-half inch. Encourage children to chew food well. Supervise meal times. Insist that children sit down while eating. Children should never run, walk, play, or lie down with food in their mouths. Be aware of older children's actions. Many choking incidents are caused when an older child gives a dangerous toy or food to a younger child.

Drowning is another leading cause of death in children. Drowning is when a child has been under water and is not breathing. Never leave a child alone in or near a tub, pail, toilet, or pool of water. A child can drown in less than 2 inches of water. See

Keep items that are choking hazards away from babies and young children. These include:

▶ Coins

▶ Buttons

▶ Toys with small parts

▶ Toys that can fit entirely in a child's mouth

▶ Small balls, marbles

▶ Balloons

▶ Small hair bows, barrettes, rubber bands

▶ Pen or marker caps

▶ Small button-type batteries

▶ Refrigerator magnets

▶ Pieces of dog food

Chapter 15: What Can I Do to Keep My Child Safe? for ways to keep your child safe around water. If your child has been under water and is not breathing, start chest compressions and rescue breathing until EMS arrives and takes over.

What You Should Look For

Look and listen for signs that your child is not breathing or is having trouble breathing.

When a child chokes, she may or may not be able to get some air into her lungs. A child who is not getting *any* air into her lungs won't be able to cry, talk, breathe, or cough. Her airway is completely blocked. If the object is not quickly removed, she will become unresponsive within minutes. When you ask an older child who has a blocked airway, "Can you talk?" she won't be able to answer. Someone who is choking may reach and clutch her neck as a signal that she is choking. This motion is known as the **universal distress signal** for choking (**Figure 3**).

universal distress signal The hands around the throat is the universal distress signal for choking.

A child who is choking but is able to get *some* air into her lungs will continue to breathe but will be coughing and anxious. Coughing is the body's way of removing what feels like a foreign object. This feeling occurs when there is swelling, irritation, or mucus anywhere in the airway. When there is an object in the airway, forceful coughing is more effective than anything you can do.

Children who are having trouble breathing may have signs of breathing problems. Here are some signs that you should look for:

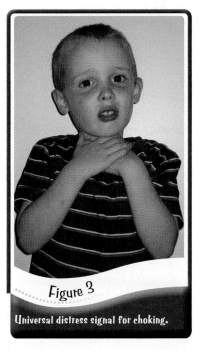

Figure 3

Universal distress signal for choking.

Breathing Effort

Normal breathing doesn't require any effort. Look for signs that the child is making an effort to breathe. You may see her nostrils flare (get bigger) each time she tries to breathe air in (**Figure 4**). She is trying to get as much air in as possible. Another sign is when the child's abdomen or chest is moving more than normal with each breath. You may see "sucking in" around the ribs. **Head bobbing**, when a child's head bobs up and down with each breath, is another serious sign.

head bobbing When a child's head bobs up and down with each breath; a serious sign that a child is having trouble breathing.

Breathing Rate

Healthy children often breathe faster than normal when they are exercising or playing. A sick child who is still and is breathing faster than normal may have a problem. A strange breathing pattern is another sign of trouble breathing.

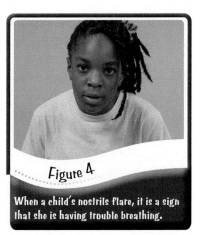

Figure 4

When a child's nostrils flare, it is a sign that she is having trouble breathing.

Keep the following foods away from children younger than 4 years:

▶ Hot dogs

▶ Nuts and seeds

▶ Chunks of meat or cheese

▶ Whole grapes

▶ Hard or sticky candy

▶ Popcorn

▶ Chunks of peanut butter

▶ Chunks of raw vegetables

▶ Chewing gum

Breathing Sounds

Normal breathing is quiet. You don't hear any unusual sounds when your child breathes in and out. Any of the following signs may mean that your child is having trouble breathing:

wheezing A whistling or squeaking sound that you hear when the child breathes out. This sound is caused by swelling or something blocking the small tubes in the lungs. Wheezing can come on suddenly. It can be a sign of an asthma attack.

snoring A rough or rattling sound with a low pitch that may be a sign that a child is having trouble breathing.

grunting Noises that a child makes when trying to breathe better; may be a sign of trouble breathing.

- **Wheezing**—A whistling or squeaking sound that you hear when the child breathes out. This sound is caused by swelling or something blocking the small tubes in the lungs. Wheezing can come on suddenly. It can be a sign of an asthma attack. If your child has asthma, your medical provider may prescribe medicine to help relieve wheezing. Be sure to know the correct way to use the medicine.

- **Snoring**—A rough or rattling sound with a low pitch. You hear it when the child breathes in.

- **Grunting**—The child makes little grunting noises each time he breathes out. He is trying to breathe better.

- **Gurgling**—You may hear gurgling or bubbling sounds when the child breathes.
- **Seal-like cough**—A barking "seal-like" cough may be a sign of croup.

Position

A child who is having trouble breathing may not want to lie down. He may be more comfortable sitting upright. Sometimes a child tries to get more air into his lungs by leaning forward in either the **sniffing position** or the **tripod position**.

- **Sniffing position**—The child leans forward and looks like he is sniffing a flower.
- **Tripod position**—The child leans forward with his arms straight. He usually props his hands on top of his knees.

Voice or Cry

The child's voice is weak, hoarse, or muffled. He can only say a few words at a time.

Anxiety

The child who is having trouble breathing may be very anxious or afraid.

Drooling

In a child who is having trouble breathing, **drooling** does not have anything to do with teething. The child drools because he can't swallow saliva due to something blocking his throat. Another cause for drooling is that the child is making extra effort to breathe.

What You Should Do

For any emergency situation, follow the Six Steps of Pediatric First Aid. If your child is having trouble breathing, call EMS or your medical provider. Give first aid care for the breathing problem as described in "What You Should Do."

gurgling Bubbling noises that you might hear in a child who is having trouble breathing.

seal-like cough A barking "seal-like" cough may be a sign of croup and that the child is having trouble breathing.

sniffing position A position a child may assume when having trouble breathing; the child will raise his head slightly and lean forward as if he is sniffing a flower.

tripod position A position a child may assume when having trouble breathing; the child will lean forward with his arms straight. He usually props his hands on top of his knees.

drooling Saliva that drips from a child's mouth. In healthy babies it is often a sign of teething. A child who is having trouble breathing may drool because of something in his throat that prevents him from swallowing. Another cause for drooling is that the child is making extra effort to breathe.

23

The Six Steps of Pediatric First Aid

1 Evaluate the Situation

Take a few seconds to look around. Evaluate the situation. Make sure the surroundings are safe. Find out who is involved and what happened.

▼

2 Look and Listen for Signs of an Emergency

Look and listen for signs that your child's condition is serious or life threatening. Notice the ABCs (Appearance, Breathing, and Circulation). Always call emergency medical services (EMS) for life-threatening conditions. To call EMS, dial 911.

▼

3 Check for Problems

Take a closer look and check your child for problems. Use the "What You Should Look For" sections to guide you. Figure out what is wrong, how serious it is, and what you should do next.

▼

4 Act

Based on what is wrong, take action. Read the "What You Should Do" sections to be prepared. For a simple injury, you may only need to give first aid. For a serious condition, you may need to call EMS and give care until help arrives.

▼

5 Follow Up

Be sure to follow up. Give any care or treatment that your child might need after the event.

▼

6 Prevent

Take steps to prevent the illness or injury from happening again, if possible. Prevention is as important as first aid in caring for your child.

First Aid for a Child* (Older Than 1 Year) Who Is Responsive and Choking

Do not give first aid for choking if your child can breathe, cry, speak, or cough. A good cough is more effective than anything you can do to clear the airway.

 Ask your child if she is choking. Not being able to breathe, cough, or make a normal voice sound are signs of choking.

 If your child is still responsive, have someone call EMS as you begin first aid care. If you are alone, call EMS after providing initial first aid care.

 Give abdominal thrusts:

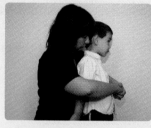

> Stand or kneel behind the child. Wrap your arms around the child at waist level.

> Place the thumb side of your fist against the child's abdomen just above the navel. Your hands will be well below the bottom tip of the breastbone and rib cage.

> Grab the fist with your other hand and press into the child's stomach with quick upward thrusts until the object is removed. Give each thrust with enough force to produce an artificial cough to help clear the airway.

> Keep giving abdominal thrusts until the object is removed, EMS takes over, or the child becomes unresponsive.

> If the child becomes unresponsive, begin CPR for a child (older than 1 year).

abdominal thrusts

A first aid technique used for a child who is choking to try to dislodge the foreign object from his airway.

*Use this first aid procedure for a child who is older than 1 year. If the child is younger than 1 year, see "First Aid for a Baby (Younger Than 1 Year) Who Is Responsive and Choking."

First Aid TIP

For a responsive child (older than 1 year) who is choking:

▶ Call EMS.*

▶ Give abdominal thrusts.

▶ Check in the mouth to see if you see a foreign object; don't try a blind finger sweep to remove any object that you cannot see.

▶ Continue until the object is coughed out, EMS takes over, or the child becomes unresponsive.

*If you are alone, give abdominal thrusts. Then call EMS.

CPR for a Child* (Older Than 1 Year) Who Is Unresponsive and Not Breathing

Rescue breathing is the technique to use when a child is not breathing. If a child is unresponsive and is not breathing or is choking and becomes unresponsive, you need to begin chest compressions followed by rescue breaths. This is called CPR.

chest compressions
Pushing hard and fast on the chest of a person who is unresponsive and not breathing.

1 CHECK FOR RESPONSIVENESS

▶ Check to see if the child is responsive. Shout, "Are you OK?" and tap the child's body. Do not use rescue breathing on a responsive child.

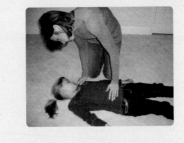

CPR for a Child (Older Than
1 Year) Who Is Unresponsive
and Not Breathing (continued)

2 CALL EMS

► Shout for help and ask someone to call 911.
► If you are alone, give 5 cycles of chest compressions and rescue breaths (about 2 minutes) then dial 911 or your local emergency number.
 − One cycle of CPR is 30 chest compressions and 2 rescue breaths.

3 GIVE CHEST COMPRESSIONS

► Place heel of one or two hands on the center of the chest. Do not press near the bottom tip of the breastbone.
► Push hard: press down on the chest 2 inches or at least ⅓ the depth of the chest.
► Push fast: press and release at a rate of at least 100 times per minute. Let the chest completely recoil (return to normal position) after each compression.

Give 30 chest compressions then alternate with 2 breaths. Continue alternating 30 chest compressions with 2 breaths until EMS takes over or until the child responds.

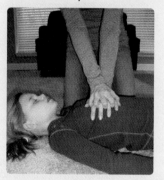

4 GIVE RESCUE BREATHS

► Open the child's airway by gently tilting the head back with one hand and lifting the chin up with other hand.
► If you see a foreign object, remove it; do not do a blind finger sweep.
► Take a normal breath (not a deep breath).

CPR for a Child* (Older Than 1 Year) Who Is Unresponsive and Not Breathing (continued)

▶ Pinch the child's nose. Breathe into the child's mouth.

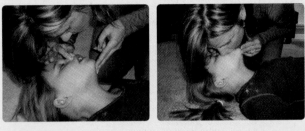

▶ Give 2 breaths, each breath for 1 second. Each breath should make the chest rise.

* Use this first aid procedure for a child who is older than 1 year. If the child is younger than 1 year, use "First Aid for a Baby (Younger Than 1 Year) Who Is Unresponsive and Not Breathing."

First Aid TIP

Using an AED

AED
An automated external defibrillator is a small, electronic device that can analyze a heart rhythm and deliver a shock to help the heart start beating again. Use an AED for a victim in cardiac arrest as soon as one is available.

An **AED (automated external defibrillator)** is used for someone who is in cardiac arrest. It is a small, electronic device that can analyze a heart rhythm and deliver a shock to help the heart start beating again. If an AED is available when you are performing CPR, it should be used. Continue chest compressions and rescue breathing while someone else turns on the AED and attaches the pads. Many AEDs are designed to be used for children under the age of 8 years old as well as for children older than 8 years and adults. These AEDs come with child pads and adult pads. Use child pads for a child. Use adult pads for a child older than 8 years old. Once the pads are attached, follow the instructions given by the AED. The AED will check the child's heart rhythm and decide whether or not to deliver a shock. Be sure that no one is touching the child when a shock is delivered. Immediately after a shock is delivered, start chest compressions and rescue breathing again.

It is very important to minimize interruptions of rescue breathing and chest compressions.

To learn more about how to use an AED, take a community class in CPR for parents and caregivers. A class will give you a chance to practice CPR and use an AED. Any attempts at CPR when needed are better than nothing. But a child's chance of recovery is greatly improved with high-quality CPR.

First Aid for a Baby* (Younger Than 1 Year) Who Is Responsive and Choking

Do not give first aid for choking if your baby can breathe, cry, speak, or cough. A good cough is more effective than anything you can do to clear the airway.

 Decide if your baby is choking. Not being able to breathe, cough, or make a normal voice sound are signs of choking.

 If your baby is still responsive, have someone call EMS as you begin first aid care. If you are alone, call EMS after providing 2 minutes of first aid care.

 Hold the baby's head and neck with one hand by supporting the baby's jaw between your thumb and fingers.

 Give 5 back blows. Using the heel of your hand, give 5 quick, sharp back blows between the baby's shoulder blades.

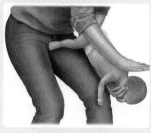

 Turn the baby over. Use both hands and forearms (one on the back and one on the front of the baby's body) to firmly hold the body as you turn the baby over. Once turned on his back, the baby should be resting on your arm, with your arm against your thigh. The baby's head should be lower than your trunk.

Give 5 chest compressions. To do this, place two fingers of one hand on the center of the breastbone just below an imaginary line drawn between the baby's nipples. Give 5 chest compressions, one right after the other. Push the breastbone down 1½ inches or at least ⅓ the depth of the chest.

back blows
A first aid technique used for a baby who is choking to try to dislodge the foreign object from his airway; back blows are alternated with chest compressions.

chest compressions
A first aid technique used for a baby who is choking to try to dislodge the foreign object from his airway; chest compressions are alternated with back blows.

First Aid for a Baby* (Younger Than 1 Year) Who Is Responsive and Choking (continued)

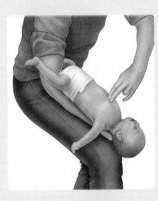

 Alternate back blows and chest compressions until the object is coughed up, EMS takes over, or the baby becomes unresponsive.

8 If the baby becomes unresponsive, begin CPR for a baby (younger than 1 year).

---

*Use this first aid procedure for a baby who is younger than 1 year. If the child is older than 1 year, see "First Aid for a Child (Older Than 1 Year) Who Is Responsive and Choking."

First Aid TIP

For a responsive baby (younger than 1 year) who is choking:

▷ Call EMS.*

▷ Give 5 back blows.

▷ Turn the baby over.

▷ Give 5 chest compressions.

▷ Check in the baby's mouth to see if you see a foreign object; don't try a blind finger sweep to remove an object that you cannot see.

▷ Continue until the object is coughed up, EMS takes over, or the baby becomes unresponsive.

---

*If you are alone, give 2 minutes of back blows and chest compressions. Then call EMS.

CPR for a Baby*
(Younger Than 1 Year)
Who Is Unresponsive and Not Breathing

Rescue breathing is the technique to use when a baby is not breathing. If a baby is unresponsive and is not breathing or is choking and becomes unresponsive, you need to begin chest compressions followed by rescue breathing. This is called CPR.

 CHECK FOR RESPONSIVENESS

► Check to see if the baby is responsive. Shout, "Are you OK?" and tap the baby's body. Do not use rescue breathing on a responsive baby.

 CALL EMS

► Shout for help and ask someone to call 911.

► If you are alone, give 5 cycles of chest compressions and rescue breaths, then dial 911 or your local emergency number.

– One cycle of CPR is 30 chest compressions and 2 rescue breaths.

③ GIVE CHEST COMPRESSIONS

► Place two fingers of one hand on the center of the breastbone just below an imaginary line drawn between the baby's nipples.

► Push hard: press down on the chest 1½ inches or at least ⅓ the depth of the chest.

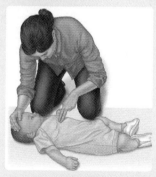

► Push fast: press and release at a rate of at least 100 times per minute. Let the chest completely recoil (return to normal) after each compression.

Give 30 chest compressions then alternate with 2 breaths. Keep alternating 30 chest compressions with 2 rescue breaths for 5 cycles of CPR. If no one has called for EMS, do it now. It is okay to carry the infant to the phone with you. Continue until EMS takes over or until the baby responds.

CPR for a Baby* (Younger Than
1 Year) Who Is Unresponsive
and Not Breathing (continued)

4 GIVE RESCUE BREATHS

▶ Open the baby's airway: gently tilt the head back with one hand, and lift the chin up with other hand.

▶ If you see a foreign object, remove it; do not do a blind finger sweep.

▶ Take a normal breath (not a deep breath).

▶ Seal your mouth over the baby's mouth and nose.

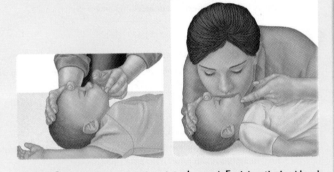

▶ Give 2 breaths, each rescue breath for 1 second. Each breath should make the chest rise.

---

*Use this first aid procedure for a baby younger than 1 year. If the child is older than 1 year, use "First Aid for a Child (Older Than 1 Year) Who Is Unresponsive and Not Breathing."

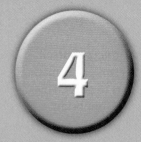

Controlling Infection, Bleeding, and Swelling

● Controlling Infection

Introduction

Infections are caused by viruses, bacteria, and other germs. Infections can be passed from one person to another. Knowing how germs spread and how to protect against infection is an important part of first aid.

What You Should Know

To control the spread of infection, take steps to protect yourself, your child, and others from exposure to germs. Germs can spread disease. Germs can enter a cut in the skin and start to grow. This can cause a wound to get infected. Good hygiene is important to help prevent the spread of germs and control infection.

body fluids All fluids that come from the body. These include urine, feces, saliva, blood, and vomit.

Take special precautions when handling blood and body fluids. **Body fluids** include urine, feces, and vomit. When body fluids contact an object that others might touch, remove germs by cleaning with detergent and rinsing with water. This will help remove the source of infection. Some germs will still be there, however, even though you can't see them. Use a sanitizer to get rid of those. This two-step process will help prevent infection from body fluids. See "What You Should Do: How to Clean Up Body Fluids to Prevent the Spread of Germs."

protective gloves
Nonporous gloves, such as disposable medical gloves or rubber dishwashing gloves.

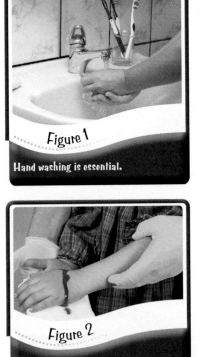

Figure 1

Hand washing is essential.

Figure 2

Disposable medical gloves can protect you and your child against germs.

Hand washing after cleaning and sanitizing is essential (**Figure 1**). You should wash your hands carefully after contact with body fluids, even if you wore **protective gloves**.

Health authorities recommend wearing protective gloves when giving first aid care to a sick or injured child (**Figure 2**). Disposable medical gloves are inexpensive and good to have in your first aid supplies. Gloves protect you and your child from germs. They also help prevent the spread of germs. You also can use rubber household gloves to protect your hands when cleaning up body fluids.

Remember to take steps to control the spread of germs. This will protect you and your family from exposure to diseases.

First Aid TIP

Control the spread of germs and prevent infection by reducing contact with germs. The following can help:

▶ Wear protective gloves that are nonporous when coming in contact with body fluids (Figure 2). Examples of protective gloves are disposable medical gloves and rubber household gloves.

▶ Use disposable towels, such as paper towels, for cleaning up and sanitizing surfaces.

▶ Select nonporous surfaces for areas that will be exposed to body fluids, such as a changing table. You want to be able to clean and sanitize the surface.

▶ Use plastic bags to store contaminated articles until they can be thrown away or sanitized.

Always wash your hands well after contact with body fluids. This is important even if you wore protective gloves.

What You Should Look For

When a child has been injured, look for places where the skin has been cut. Look for bleeding, bruising, swelling, or pain. These may be signs of tissue injury. Tissue injury may come from a blow. It also may be caused by a force that twists or pinches a body part. One example of a tissue injury is a sprain.

Look to see if you have cuts or open sores on your own hands. If so, you might get an infection from contact with germs on surfaces or from body fluids. You will need to protect yourself from infection. Keep cuts or sores covered with clean bandages. Wear protective gloves when handling body fluids.

What You Should Do

Reducing the number of germs in a cut or wound helps prevent infection. First, control bleeding. Then, clean the wound with soap and running water as soon as possible. This important first aid step removes dirt and germs. The sooner germs are rinsed out of a wound, the better. Promptly rinse all wounds, except for wounds that are bleeding freely or nosebleeds.

Did You Know?

Awareness for protection from body fluids came about because of the HIV/AIDS virus. HIV is transmitted through body fluids. It is mostly transmitted through sexual intercourse, breastfeeding, childbirth, sharing of needles, and blood transfusions. HIV is not transmitted by saliva, tears, sweat, feces, or urine. HIV is not transmitted by hugging, kissing, shaking hands, insect bites, or sharing toilets with an HIV-positive person.

Anyone with HIV is considered to be HIV positive. People who are HIV positive are never "cured" but do not always develop AIDS. They can lead normal lives and may never have complications.

Germs grow very quickly in a wound. They can soon overwhelm the body's defenses against infection.

Keep germs from spreading by properly cleaning up body fluids such as urine, feces, and vomit.

How to Clean Up Body Fluids to Prevent the Spread of Germs

 When you need to clean up body fluids, wear protective gloves. Try to use disposable cleaning tools, such as paper towels. Avoid spreading the spilled body fluid.

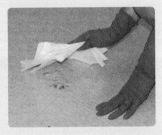

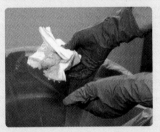 Put disposable cleaning tools, such as paper towels, in a plastic-lined trashcan for disposal. Put tools that you need to sanitize later, such as a mop, in another plastic-lined trashcan or pail.

 Use detergent to clean all surfaces that came in contact with the body fluid.

Rinse cleaned surfaces with water.

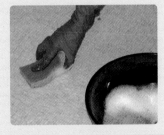

Apply a sanitizing solution. Follow the instructions on the label. (Make your own sanitizing solution by mixing one-fourth cup of household bleach with 1 gallon of water, or 1 tablespoon of bleach to 1 quart of water. Leave this solution in contact with the surface for at least 2 minutes.)

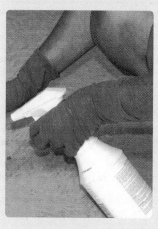

 Put the cleaning material that you used to wipe up the sanitizing solution in a plastic-lined trashcan for disposal.

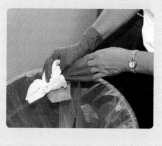

 # Bleeding

What You Should Know

When the skin is cut, blood vessels are broken. This is why a cut bleeds. Some blood vessels bleed more than others. Cuts in certain types of blood vessels are more serious than in other types. Deep cuts are more serious than shallow ones. Understanding more about blood vessels will help you take the best first aid steps (**Table 1**). To

Table 1 Blood Vessels

Type of Blood Vessel	More Information	First Aid Tips
Capillaries	These are tiny blood vessels. There are thousands throughout the body.	Bleeding is easy to control. Apply direct pressure to stop bleeding from capillaries.
Veins	Veins are located close to the surface of the skin.	Veins can bleed heavily. Apply direct pressure to control bleeding from veins.
Arteries	Arteries are large, deep blood vessels. Large amounts of blood can be lost from arteries in a short amount of time.	Bleeding from an artery may be life threatening. Apply direct pressure and call EMS.

capillaries Tiny blood vessels located throughout the body. There are thousands of them. Bleeding is easy to control from capillaries.

veins Veins are located close to the surface of the skin. Veins can bleed heavily.

arteries Large, deep, and well-protected blood vessels. Arteries carry blood away from the heart to all parts of the body. Large amounts of blood can be lost from arteries in a short amount of time. Bleeding from an artery may be life threatening.

direct pressure Pressing directly over a wound to stop bleeding, usually with a sterile dressing or clean, dry cloth.

dressing A clean covering placed over a wound. A gauze pad can be used as a dressing.

stop or control bleeding, apply pressure. Use a sterile dressing or clean, dry cloth to press on the wound. This is called **direct pressure**. Wear medical gloves if available.

Some parts of the body have more blood vessels than others. For example, the head and face have more blood vessels in a given area than the finger. That is why a cut on the head or face bleeds more than a cut on a finger.

You may need to apply a dressing or bandage. A **dressing** is a clean covering placed over a wound (**Figure 3**). A gauze pad can be used as a dressing. A **bandage** holds the dressing in place. It also can be used to apply pressure to help control bleeding (**Figure 4**). Adhesive tape and rolls of gauze are often used as bandages. An **adhesive bandage** is a combination of a dressing and a bandage. All of these come in a variety of sizes.

An injury that is deep in the chest, abdomen, or brain may cause bleeding far below the skin. This type of injury is called **internal bleeding**. Symptoms vary and depend upon the type of injury. Usually, a child with internal bleeding feels severe pain and looks very sick. If you suspect internal bleeding, call EMS right away. Try to keep your child calm while waiting for EMS to arrive.

If the skin is broken, the wound is called an **open wound**. Common types of open wounds are scrapes, cuts, broken blisters, punctures, and nosebleeds.

- A **scrape** occurs when the top layer of skin has been rubbed off (**Figure 5**). Children often get scrapes on their elbows or knees. Scrapes usually don't bleed very much but can get infected. Because nerve endings just under the skin may be exposed, scrapes can be quite painful.
- A **cut** may be jagged or smooth (**Figure 6**). It may be shallow, like a paper cut, or deep. Cuts may be large or small.
- A **blister** is fluid that collects in a bubble under the skin. Blisters can be small or large. The fluid inside a blister is sterile if the skin is not broken.
- A **puncture** is a small hole made in the skin. It may either be deep or shallow. Puncture wounds usually don't bleed very much. Punctures have a high risk of infection because it is hard to wash the germs out. An example of a puncture wound is a splinter.
- A **nosebleed** is bleeding from the nose. Nosebleeds occur more often in the winter. This is due to respiratory infections and dry air, which may cause itching and picking of the nose. Blowing the nose too hard or hitting the nose can cause nosebleeds also.

bandage Holds the dressing in place. It also can be used to apply pressure to help control bleeding. Adhesive tape and rolls of gauze are often used as bandages.

adhesive bandage Combination of a dressing and a bandage.

internal bleeding Bleeding in tissues far below the skin caused by an injury that is deep in the chest, abdomen, or brain.

open wound Broken skin as a result of an injury. Common types of open wounds are scrapes, cuts, broken blisters, punctures, and nosebleeds.

scrape An open wound that occurs when the top layer of skin is rubbed off. Because nerve endings just under the skin may be exposed, scrapes can be quite painful.

cut An incision in the skin, which may be jagged or smooth. It may be shallow, like a paper cut, or deep. Cuts may be large or small.

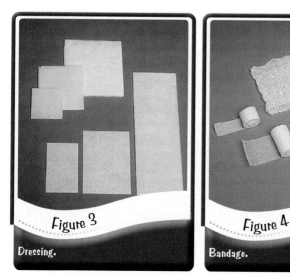

Figure 3

Dressing.

Figure 4

Bandage.

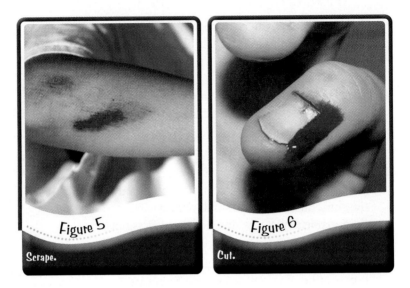

Figure 5

Scrape.

Figure 6

Cut.

First Aid TIP

Most bleeding in children is not life threatening. Usually bleeding from small blood vessels stops quickly. Don't panic when you see what seems to be a lot of blood coming from a cut anywhere on the head or face. Because blood is a bright red color, a little blood may look like a larger volume than it really is. Bleeding that does not stop by itself within a minute or so needs first aid care. You want to stop the bleeding before larger amounts of blood are lost.

Another type of open wound that is rare is when a part of the body has been torn or cut off. Call EMS right away and control the bleeding.

What You Should Look For

1 Look carefully to see where the blood is coming from. A child who has a small cut on the inside of his lip may have blood on his face, lips, tongue, shirt, and hands. Until you find the source of the blood, you might think that the cut is much bigger than it actually is.

2 Check if the cut is still bleeding or if the flow of blood has stopped.

3 Carefully watch a child who has had a hard fall. If he is in pain or looks very sick, he might have internal bleeding.

What You Should Do

For any medical situation, follow the Six Steps of Pediatric First Aid. If your child is bleeding heavily or you can't get the bleeding to stop, call EMS. Give first aid care until EMS providers arrive and take over.

Some dressings have a plastic back to keep blood from leaking through to the outside. Small plastic-backed dressings can be serious choking hazards for children younger than 3 years old. A young child may take the plastic-backed dressing off a wound and put it in his mouth. If the plastic dressing gets positioned across the airway, the child may not be able to breathe. Avoid plastic-backed dressings for children younger than 3 years old. Use fabric bandages and dressings instead.

The Six Steps of Pediatric First Aid

1 Evaluate the Situation

Take a few seconds to look around. Evaluate the situation. Make sure the surroundings are safe. Find out who is involved and what happened.

▼

2 Look and Listen for Signs of an Emergency

Look and listen for signs that your child's condition is serious or life threatening. Notice the ABCs (Appearance, Breathing, and Circulation). Always call emergency medical services (EMS) for life-threatening conditions. To call EMS, dial 911.

▼

3 Check for Problems

Take a closer look and check your child for problems. Use the "What You Should Look For" sections to guide you. Figure out what is wrong, how serious it is, and what you should do next.

▼

 **4** **Act**

Based on what is wrong, take action. Read the "What You Should Do" sections to be prepared. For a simple injury, you may only need to give first aid. For a serious condition, you may need to call EMS and give care until help arrives.

▼

 5 **Follow Up**

Be sure to follow up. Give any care or treatment that your child might need after the event.

▼

6 **Prevent**

Take steps to prevent the illness or injury from happening again, if possible. Prevention is as important as first aid in caring for your child.

First Aid Care for Minor Scrapes and Cuts

1 Press on the wound with a sterile dressing or clean, dry cloth to stop bleeding. Wear medical gloves if available.

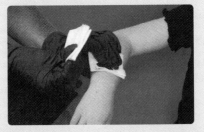

2 If bleeding is from an arm or leg, raise the arm or leg while still pressing on the wound. Don't raise an arm or leg that is broken.

3 Wash a shallow wound with clean, running water. Carefully wash the area around the wound with soap and a soft wash cloth. Try to keep soap out of the wound to avoid irritation. Don't use hydrogen peroxide or alcohol to clean a wound unless your medical provider tells you to.

(4) Apply a bandage.

(5) If the scrape or cut is very dirty, your child may need a tetanus booster shot. Check with a medical provider if your child's last tetanus shot was more than 5 years ago.

First Aid TIP

Have the following wounds evaluated by a medical provider as soon as possible:

▶ A wound that will not stay closed by itself

▶ A wound that needs 5 minutes of constant direct pressure to stop the bleeding

▶ A cut longer than one-half inch

Some wounds may need stitches, tape, or some other method to help healing. These need to be applied as soon as possible—usually within 6 hours of the injury. Prompt and proper cleaning, followed by closing of an open wound, reduces the risk of infection. This also helps the wound heal faster and reduces the chance of scarring.

First Aid TIP

A child can suck on a popsicle to apply cold and pressure to a cut on the lip or tongue. This is also good for an injured tooth.

First Aid Care for Deep Scrapes, Cuts, and Open Wounds

 Press on the wound with a sterile dressing or clean, dry cloth to control bleeding. Wear medical gloves if available. Usually bleeding will stop after 1 to 2 minutes. If bleeding is easy to control, clean and bandage the wound as you would for a minor scrape or cut.

 If bleeding is from an arm or leg, raise the arm or leg while still pressing on the wound. Don't raise an arm or leg that is broken.

 If bleeding is hard to control, keep applying pressure for at least 5 minutes. If blood seeps through the cloth while you apply pressure, don't replace it with a clean cloth. Put another cloth on top. Removing the first cloth might disturb the clot that is forming. A clot will plug up the blood vessel and stop the bleeding.

 Don't try to clean a deep wound or put medicine on it. A deep wound needs to be cleaned by a medical provider.

Ⓢ If bleeding doesn't stop after 5 minutes, call EMS or get medical care. For very serious bleeding, you can try to slow the bleeding by applying pressure to a pressure point.

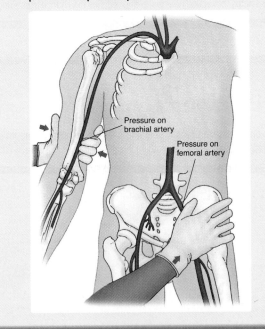

Pressure on brachial artery

Pressure on femoral artery

First Aid Care for Deep
Scrapes, Cuts, and Open Wounds
(continued)

 6 If the scrape or cut is very dirty, your child may need a tetanus booster shot. Check with a medical provider if your child's last tetanus shot was more than 5 years ago.

First Aid TIP

A child who suffers a serious injury and loses a lot of blood can go into shock. Some signs of shock are dizziness, fast breathing, and fast heartbeat. Another sign is cool, moist, pale skin. A child in shock may be very anxious. Try to keep the child calm while waiting for EMS to come. Care for shock by laying the child down on his back. Raise his legs 8 to 10 inches. Cover the child with blankets to keep him warm.

First Aid Care
for Blisters

 1 Protect blisters with a bandage. Don't "pop" a blister. You want to keep the blister from opening so that the injured tissue underneath can heal.

2 Take your child to a medical provider if a blister is larger than a quarter.

 3 If the blister opens, clean it with water. Care for it in the same way you would a minor scrape or cut.

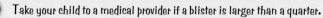

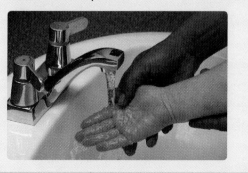

First Aid Care for Punctures, Including Splinters

 Pull out a small object that you can grasp easily with clean tweezers, such as a wood splinter or a staple. Get medical care if you cannot get a small object out easily or if it is too deep. Call EMS if the object is large, such as a knife or stick stuck deep below the skin. Don't try to pull the object out. If you need to, apply a bandage so that the object doesn't move around. You want to keep it from doing more damage while you are waiting for medical care.

 Soak the wound in clean water.

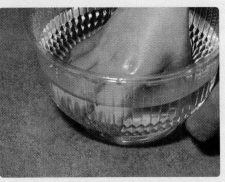

 If the object is out, soak the wound again in clean water.

 Leave the wound without a bandage, if possible. If it needs a bandage, put the bandage on loosely.

 If the object was very dirty, your child may need a tetanus booster shot. Check with a medical provider if your child's last tetanus shot was more than 5 years ago.

Tetanus is a disease that is sometimes called "lock-jaw." Bacteria that can cause tetanus live in the soil, in dust, and in human and animal feces. These bacteria enter the body through a dirty wound and cause tetanus. This disease causes strong spasms in the back, legs, arms, and jaw (lockjaw). Tetanus is usually fatal. Routine and periodic tetanus vaccinations have made most people in the United States immune to tetanus. Vaccination teaches the immune system of the body to develop protection against tetanus. Children should get routine tetanus shots at 2 months, 4 months, 6 months, 12 to 15 months, and 4 to 6 years old. Tetanus booster shots should be given every 10 years from then on throughout life. A child will only need an extra shot at the time of injury if a wound is very dirty and if it has been at least 5 years since the last booster.

tetanus A fatal disease caused when bacteria that live in the soil, in dust, and in human and animal feces enter the body through a wound. This disease causes strong spasms in the back, legs, arms, and jaw (lockjaw). Vaccinations protect against this disease.

First Aid Care for Nosebleeds

 Keep the child sitting up.

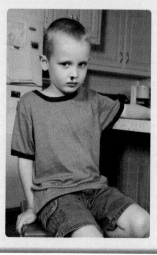

If the child can do so easily, have him gently blow his nose before you apply pressure as described in the next step. Having the child blow his nose right before you apply pressure is helpful. There will be less blood in the nose to cause problems after the bleeding stops.

 Use the thumb and a finger of one hand to pinch the soft parts of the nose together.

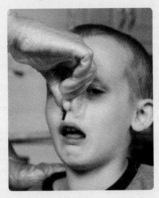

 Gently press the pinched nose against the bones of the face.

 Hold that position for a full 5 minutes. Don't peek to see if bleeding has stopped.

 At the same time, apply ice to the child's nose and cheeks if you can. Use a plastic bag of ice or a package of frozen vegetables wrapped in a cloth. (Don't apply ice or frozen vegetables directly to the child's skin.)

 After 5 minutes of pressure, gently release the nose, little by little. You want to avoid a sudden rush of blood back into the nose. That might make the nose bleed again. If bleeding does start again, pinch the nose and apply pressure as before. Hold the pressure for more than 5 minutes this time.

 Have the child do a quiet activity, such as reading, for at least 30 minutes after the nosebleed stops.

 Don't have the child blow his nose after the nosebleed stops. Blowing the nose could dislodge the clot. Having the child blow his nose right before you apply pressure is helpful. This way there will be less blood in the nose after the bleeding stops. Large amounts of blood left in the nose may form scabs, which are itchy. The child may pick at the scabs and start the bleeding again.

Call EMS or get medical care if a nosebleed cannot be controlled.

Did You Know?

The air tends to be very dry in desert climates and in the winter months in cold climates. The air is dry in air-conditioned rooms also. Adding moisture to dry air with a humidifier or vaporizer helps to reduce the risk of nosebleeds. When nosebleeds are a problem, some medical providers recommend the use of saline nasal mist spray three times per day. They also recommend putting petroleum jelly in the child's nasal openings. These measures help protect the delicate nasal tissue from harsh, dry air.

Swelling

What You Should Know

Sometimes an injury will crush small blood vessels but will not break the skin. Bleeding from blood vessels under the skin is called a **bruise**. Active children often get bruises (**Figure 7**). At first, a bruise looks red and swollen. Then it gradually turns blue or purple. As the blood is absorbed over the next few days, the area turns yellow and fades as it heals.

bruise Bleeding from blood vessels under the skin.

Sometimes injuries will cause swelling. Swelling or bruising can be a sign of a **crush injury**. Crush injuries happen when a body part is squeezed or twisted between two hard surfaces. Automobile crashes can

crush injury An injury that results from squeezing or twisting a body part between two hard surfaces. Automobile crashes and hard falls can cause crush injuries.

49

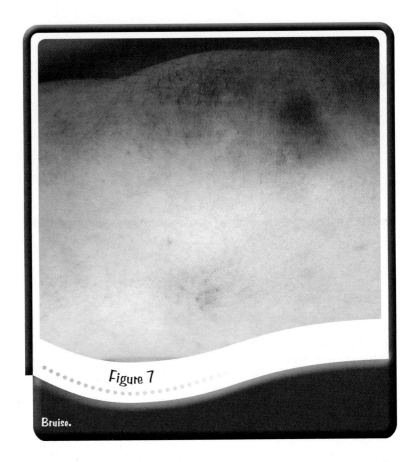

Figure 7

Bruise.

cause crush injuries. A crush injury can happen if a heavy door slams on a child's hand. A hard fall can cause a crush injury. Always get medical care if you think your child has a crush injury.

What You Should Look For

- Check to see what caused the injury.
- Compare the injured part of the body with the same body part on the opposite side to see if there is swelling.
- Touch the skin to see if the skin feels tight.
- Look for skin that is red or bruised over the injured area.
- If you suspect a crush injury, get medical care right away.

50

First Aid Care for Bruises and Swelling

 1 To control swelling, apply a cold pack wrapped in a thin cloth. You also can use ice or a package of frozen vegetables wrapped in a cloth. (Don't apply ice or frozen vegetables directly to the child's skin. This can cause damage to the tissues.) You can use stretchy rolled gauze or an elastic bandage to hold a cold pack in place.

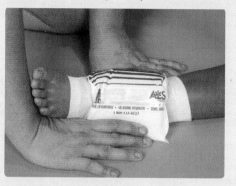

 2 Call EMS or get medical care if your child keeps having pain or swelling.

3 Call EMS or get medical care if you think your child could have a crush injury.

4 Put pressure on a bruised or swollen area by wrapping it with stretchy rolled gauze or an elastic bandage. Leave the tips of the child's fingers and toes exposed so that you can tell if the bandage is too tight. Check often to make sure the fingers or toes are still a normal skin color and feel warm to the touch.

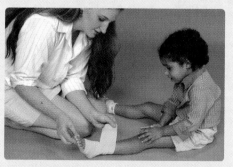

 5 Raise the injured arm or leg unless you suspect a broken bone or a spinal injury. Moving a child with a broken bone or a spinal injury can cause more injury.

Bone, Joint, and Muscle Injuries

● Bone, Joint, and Muscle Injuries

Introduction

The bones and joints of young children are generally more flexible than those of adults. Children rarely get hurt while stretching, bending, or running. Young children's joints, however, are more easily dislocated than adults'. Dislocation of the elbow is more common in children. Because children are active and not always cautious, they sometimes get broken bones and bruises. Injuries to the spine can be very serious. Try not to move a child who has fallen because a spinal injury is possible.

What You Should Know

Any bone in the body can be broken. A broken bone is sometimes called a **fracture**. A fracture can be a partial break or a complete break in the bone. When a bone breaks, the muscles, nerves, and blood vessels around the bone can be hurt too.

fracture A broken bone.

closed fracture The skin is not broken at the location of the fracture.

Fractures can be closed or open (**Figure 1**). In a **closed fracture**, the skin is not broken at the location of the fracture. In an **open fracture**, there is an open wound over the fracture. The wound can be caused by the broken bone cutting through the skin or from the

open fracture There is an open wound over the fracture. The wound can be caused by the bone breaking through the skin. It also can be caused from the force that broke the bone.

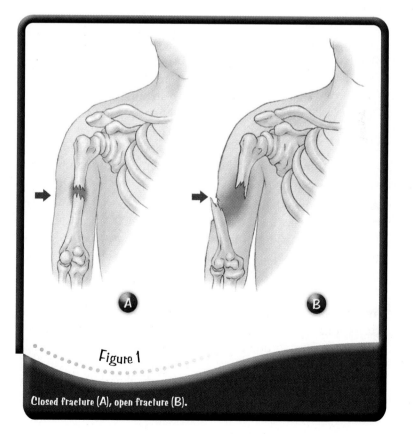

Figure 1

Closed fracture (A), open fracture (B).

force that broke the bone. Blood loss in both open and closed fractures is the same, but you will see more blood in an open fracture. Open fractures have a greater chance of infection.

Fractures are common in children. Fortunately, children's bones heal quickly. Although the bone usually heals completely, that part of the body may not grow normally. The flexibility to move through a full range of motion also may be affected.

dislocation The separation of a bone from a joint.

A **dislocation** is the separation of a bone from a joint. In children, dislocations often happen to fingers and elbows. These are not always obvious. It takes only a small amount of force to dislocate a child's bone. A quick tug on a child's hand to prevent him from running into the street can be enough to dislocate his elbow. Always pick up babies and young children by lifting them from under their arms. Never pick up a child by his hands or wrists (**Figure 2**).

Sometimes a dislocated bone will go back into the socket by itself right away. Often a medical provider will need to return the bone to its proper position. If the bone stays dislocated, the joint will not be able to move. This will cause pain.

sprain An injury to a ligament caused when the ligament is stretched beyond its limit.

ligaments The tissues that hold the joints together.

strain An injury to a muscle caused when the muscle is stretched beyond its limit.

A **sprain** is an injury to a ligament. **Ligaments** are thick tissues that hold the joints together. Sprains happen when ligaments are stretched beyond their limits. A **strain** is an injury to muscles. Strains happen when muscles are stretched beyond their limits. Sprains and strains don't happen often to young children. But as a child's joints and muscles become more like an adult's, sprains and strains become more common.

At the time of an injury, most children do not want to move the body part that has a fractured bone or hurt joint or muscle. These injuries cause pain and muscle spasm. The instinct is to hold the injured body part very still. Another way children "splint" their own injury is by holding the injured body part close against their body.

You do not need to figure out whether your child has a fracture, dislocation, sprain, or strain. First aid is the same for any of these injuries. It is important to recognize when your child might have an injury that could be serious. Then the best action is to keep the injured part from moving until a medical provider can evaluate your child.

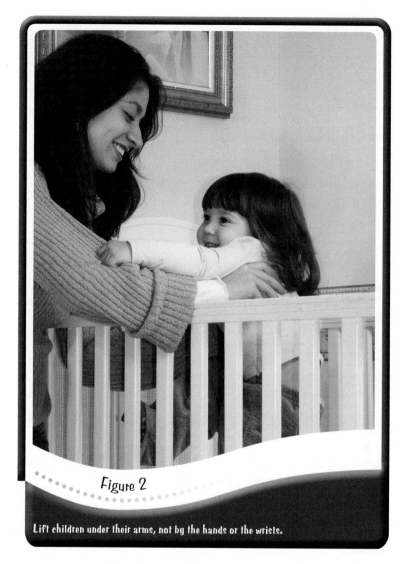

Figure 2

Lift children under their arms, not by the hands or the wrists.

What You Should Look For

You may suspect an injury to your child's bones, joints, or muscles when you first assess the situation. As you figure out what happened, you will learn if your child has fallen or been struck by some force. You will notice if your child is holding a body part very still in an unnatural way.

Often you can tell from a distance if your child is in pain. Your child may complain of pain at the site that is bruised or bleeding. Even if the child is crying, you can try to get him to point to where

55

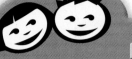

Keep Your Child Safe from Falls

▸ Use gates at the bottom and top of stairs.

▸ Install operable window guards on all windows above the first floor.

▸ Don't leave a baby alone on a changing table, bed, sofa, or chair—even for a moment.

▸ Keep the crib side up. Even if your baby is not rolling over or pulling up, there's always a first time.

▸ Secure elevated surfaces, such as balconies.

▸ Don't use a baby walker that can move across the floor. A baby may tip the walker over, fall out of it, or fall down stairs.

▸ Check the surface under play equipment. There should be cushioning material that will absorb the force of a fall, such as a safety rubber mat. Other acceptable materials are 12 inches of sand, sawdust, or wood chips.

it hurts. Asking the child to point to the spot that hurts helps distract him from the pain. This also will help you avoid jumping to a wrong conclusion about which body part has been hurt. It can be hard to figure out where the injury is when a child is crying or refusing to move. The child may be holding an uninjured part to keep the injured part still. Children figure out within seconds that not moving an injured part reduces the pain.

DOTS Memory aid for assessing bone, joint, and muscle injuries: Deformity, Open injury, Tenderness, Swelling.

When dealing with bone, joint, and muscle injuries, use **DOTS** (Deformity, Open injury, Tenderness, and Swelling) as a memory aid to help figure out what is wrong and how serious it is (**Table 1**).

deformity An abnormal shape caused by a broken bone.

Sometimes a break in the bone causes an unnatural shape or bend in part of the body. This unnatural appearance is called a **deformity**. To detect a deformity, compare the injured body part with the side that isn't injured. An injured area may be tender and sensitive to touch.

Table 1 DOTS

D	Deformity	Look for an abnormal shape caused by a broken bone
O	Open injuries or wounds	Look for bleeding and breaks in the skin
T	Tenderness	Check for areas that are sensitive to touch
S	Swelling	Look for areas that look larger than usual

Remember that loss of movement is a sign that a bone, joint, or muscle may be injured. The child may be able to move the injured part slightly but not have full range of motion. When bones, joints, or muscles are injured, blood and other fluids collect around the injury. This buildup of fluid causes swelling.

What You Should Do

For any medical situation, follow the Six Steps of Pediatric First Aid. If your child has a bone, joint, or muscle injury, give first aid care. Based on the type of injury, you will be able to decide if you need to call EMS or get medical care.

The Six Steps of Pediatric First Aid

1 **Evaluate the Situation**

Take a few seconds to look around. Evaluate the situation. Make sure the surroundings are safe. Find out who is involved and what happened.

▼

2 **Look and Listen for Signs of an Emergency**

Look and listen for signs that your child's condition is serious or life threatening. Notice the ABCs (Appearance, Breathing, and Circulation). Always call emergency medical services (EMS) for life-threatening conditions. To call EMS, dial 911.

▼

Check for Problems

Take a closer look and check your child for problems. Use the "What You Should Look For" sections to guide you. Figure out what is wrong, how serious it is, and what you should do next.

▼

4 Act

Based on what is wrong, take action. Read the "What You Should Do" sections to be prepared. For a simple injury, you may only need to give first aid. For a serious condition, you may need to call EMS and give care until help arrives.

▼

5 Follow Up

Be sure to follow up. Give any care or treatment that your child might need after the event.

▼

6 Prevent

Take steps to prevent the illness or injury from happening again, if possible. Prevention is as important as first aid in caring for your child.

First Aid Care for Bone, Joint, and Muscle Injuries

RICE Memory aid for taking care of minor bone, joint, and muscle injuries: Rest, Ice, Compression, Elevation.

If the child can move the body part and it only hurts a little, the injury is often minor. Otherwise, a medical provider should evaluate the injury to decide what care is needed. Use the memory aid **RICE** to remember how to care for minor bone, joint, and muscle injuries.

 1 Rest: Have the child rest in a comfortable position, such as sitting or lying down. Pain is the body's way of letting us know there is a problem. If it hurts to move an injured body part, then it is best not to move it.

2 Ice: Cover the injury with a cloth and apply ice or a cold pack for 20 to 30 minutes at a time. Do this every 2 to 3 hours for the first 24 to 48 hours. This reduces pain, bleeding, and swelling. Always protect the skin by wrapping ice or a cold pack in a thin cloth. Direct contact of extreme cold on the skin can cause tissue damage. An elastic bandage is a good way to hold the ice or cold pack in place. Continuous use of ice or direct contact of ice with the skin can damage the tissue.

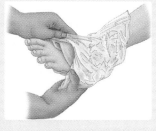

3 Compression: You can use an elastic bandage to compress the injured area. This helps keep blood and other fluids from collecting. Start a few inches below and end several inches above the injury. Wrap upward toward the heart in a spiral motion. Use firm, even pressure, making sure you do not wrap too tightly. If the child complains that his fingers or toes are cold, tingling, or numb, loosen the bandage. Remove the elastic bandage only when applying ice.

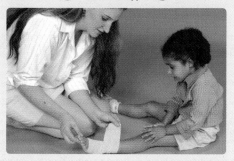

4 Elevation: Elevate the injury above the level of the heart. Place the injured limb on several pillows. This limits blood flow to the injury and reduces swelling.

Did You Know?

Who Should Splint the Injury?

splinting Keeping an injured body part from moving.

Splinting is taking steps to keep an injured body part from moving. The best action is to wait for EMS or a medical provider to splint the injured part. There are some situations, however, when a splint might be needed right away. You may need to splint a young child's injury if direct pressure is required to control bleeding. You may need to apply a splint if you must move the child before EMS arrives. Reasons to wait for EMS to splint the injured part are the following:

▶ EMS providers are trained to apply a splint quickly and safely.

▶ Someone who has only first aid training may not apply the splint in the right way. A splint that is too tight or that positions a limb incorrectly can restrict circulation.

▶ A young child in pain may not cooperate.

▶ Moving the injury during splinting can cause more pain or injury. It could cause damage to the bone, soft tissue, blood vessels, and nerves.

▶ Usually, a child will splint an injured body part himself by not moving it to avoid pain.

If an open wound is present, wear medical gloves if available. To control bleeding when there may be a bone injury, apply pressure on the tissues above or below the injury. If any bone ends are bleeding, apply pressure but make sure the ends don't move. If the bone ends move, the injury could get worse. If you need to control bleeding, splinting the injured area may help to prevent movement at the site of the injury.

After controlling bleeding, cover the wound with a sterile dressing or a large, clean cloth to keep the injured area as clean as possible.

First Aid TIP

How to Apply a Splint

It is better to wait for EMS to splint an injured body part. However, you may need to splint the injured body part to control bleeding or if you must move the child. To splint an injured body part, you can:

▶ Put it against an uninjured part of the child's body. For example, you can tape an injured finger to an uninjured finger next to it. This is called "buddy-splinting."

▶ Use a rigid object, like cardboard or folded newspaper, that is big enough to cross the joint above and below the injury. Put the rigid object against the injured body part. Use cloth or tape to hold it in place. This helps keep broken bone edges from moving.

Apply ice or cold packs wrapped in a thin cloth to reduce swelling and pain. Elevate a splinted injured arm or leg, as long as it does not cause more pain. This will help to reduce swelling and pain. Do not move anyone who might have a neck or spinal injury.

First Aid TIP

▶ Don't clean an open wound if you think that there might be a fracture.
▶ Don't give a child who might have a broken bone anything to eat or drink.
▶ Don't move anyone who might have a neck or spinal injury.

Injuries to the Spine

What You Should Know

The **spinal cord** is the bony column that surrounds and protects the nerves of the spine. A spinal injury is an injury that damages the spinal cord. The nerves of the spine allow sensation and movement throughout the body. Any serious injury to the spinal cord

spinal cord The bony column that surrounds and protects the nerves of the spine.

and nerves can cause paralysis below the injured area. **Paralysis** is a loss of feeling and movement.

Fractures of the spine are uncommon in children. However, if you suspect your child's back or neck could be injured, treat him as if he has a spinal injury. Any child who is unresponsive after an injury should be treated as if he has a spinal injury (**Figure 3**). Allowing a child with a spinal injury to sit up or moving him incorrectly can damage the nerves of the spine. This can cause paralysis and death. If you must move a child with a suspected spinal injury to keep him safe, use the shoulder drag method. See Figure 1 in *Chapter 2: Six Steps of Pediatric First Aid*.

What You Should Look For

- Doesn't respond as usual or doesn't respond at all
- Can't walk
- Can't move arms or legs
- Doesn't want to move neck
- Pain in the back or neck
- Tenderness, swelling, or bruising in the back or neck
- Head hurts and pain radiates through shoulders

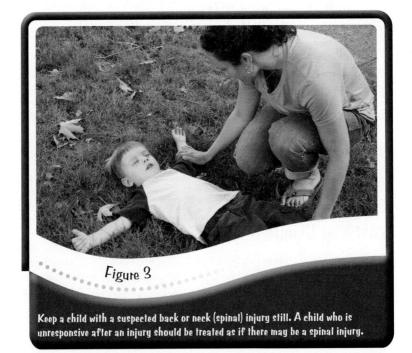

Figure 3

Keep a child with a suspected back or neck (spinal) injury still. A child who is unresponsive after an injury should be treated as if there may be a spinal injury.

Keep Your Child Safe from Sports-Related Injuries

Children as young as 4 years are playing organized sports. Every year about 4 million children go to the emergency room because of sports-related injuries. About another 8 million need to be treated for sports injuries by medical providers.

Help your child avoid sports-related injuries. Check out these important points before enrolling your child in organized sports.

▶ The coach should have education, training, and experience in organized sports for children. He should know about the health risks of training children too vigorously.

▶ All coaches, whether paid or volunteer, should have first aid skills.

▶ Children should have a complete physical examination before participating in sports.

▶ Children should know what safety equipment is needed. They should use it all the time. Make sure safety equipment fits your child properly.

▶ Playing areas should be free of dangerous debris.

▶ Warm-up and cool-down activities should always take place.

▶ Pain means that something is wrong. Children should never be told to "work through it."

Adapted from: "Sports and Injuries," The National Youth Sports Foundation for the Prevention of Athletic Injuries, Inc.

First Aid Care
for Spinal Injuries

 Make sure the child does not move and that nobody moves him. This could cause more spinal damage. Don't try to hold the child down to keep him from moving. A child with a spinal injury will either be unable to move or will find that moving hurts and will not want to move.

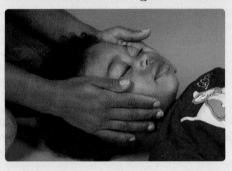

 Call EMS to transport the child to a medical facility.

Loss of Responsiveness, Fainting, and Head Injuries

Loss of Responsiveness, Fainting, and Head Injuries

Introduction

Loss of responsiveness can occur for many reasons. Some reasons are injury, severe allergic reactions, and stress. Fainting is a

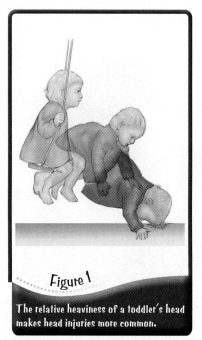

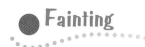

Figure 1

The relative heaviness of a toddler's head makes head injuries more common.

loss of responsiveness that is not caused by injury. Children can suffer head injuries as a result of fainting.

Head injuries are common during childhood years. For every 100,000 children younger than 5 years old, 82 will suffer a traumatic injury each year. Most of these injuries are caused by falls. Head injuries are more common in infants and toddlers. This is because a toddler's head is relatively heavy in proportion to the rest of the body (**Figure 1**). After falls, the second most common cause of head injury is motor vehicle crashes.

Low or high blood sugar in a diabetic child can be an emergency and cause loss of responsiveness.

Fainting

What You Should Know

fainting A sudden and temporary loss of responsiveness caused by a brief lack of blood and oxygen to the brain.

Fainting is a sudden loss of responsiveness that is temporary. It is caused by a brief lack of blood and oxygen to the brain. Fainting is not caused by an injury; it is a nervous system reaction to some situations. These include fear, pain, or strong emotional upset. Sometimes standing for a long time in warm conditions will cause fainting. Most of the time, fainting is not serious. Children usually recover from fainting in a few minutes without any special care.

Fainting can be prevented by lowering the head below the heart. Raising the feet above the level of the heart also can prevent fainting. These positions allow more blood to flow to the brain. Some children who faint assume an unusual position while they are unresponsive. They may bend their hands at the wrist and stiffen their legs. Unlike a seizure, there are no jerking movements.

What You Should Look For

- Lightheadedness
- Dizziness
- Nausea
- Pale skin color
- Sweating

What You Should Do

For any medical situation, follow the Six Steps of Pediatric First Aid. If your child has a loss of responsiveness, fainting, or a head injury, give first aid care. Based on the instructions in "What You Should Do," you will know if you need to call EMS or get medical care.

The Six Steps of Pediatric First Aid

1 Evaluate the Situation

Take a few seconds to look around. Evaluate the situation. Make sure the surroundings are safe. Find out who is involved and what happened.

▼

2 Look and Listen for Signs of an Emergency

Look and listen for signs that your child's condition is serious or life threatening. Notice the ABCs (Appearance, Breathing, and Circulation). Always call emergency medical services (EMS) for life-threatening conditions. To call EMS, dial 911.

▼

3 Check for Problems

Take a closer look and check your child for problems. Use the "What You Should Look For" sections to guide you. Figure out what is wrong, how serious it is, and what you should do next.

▼

4 **Act**

Based on what is wrong, take action. Read the "What You Should Do" sections to be prepared. For a simple injury, you may only need to give first aid. For a serious condition, you may need to call EMS and give care until help arrives.

▼

5 **Follow Up**

Be sure to follow up. Give any care or treatment that your child might need after the event.

▼

6 **Prevent**

Take steps to prevent the illness or injury from happening again, if possible. Prevention is as important as first aid in caring for your child.

First Aid Care for Fainting

 Lay the child on her back to prevent falling. If the child has already fainted, put the child on her back and check for breathing. If the child is not breathing, begin CPR.

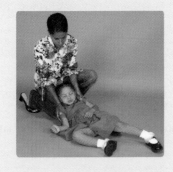

Raise the legs 8 inches to 12 inches to increase blood flow to the brain.

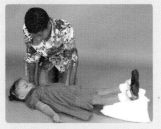

 Loosen any tight clothing.

 Call EMS if the child is unresponsive for more than a minute or so after raising her legs.

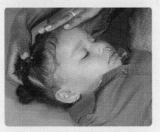

 Look for a cause of the loss of responsiveness. Consider the following:
- ► Injury
- ► Blood loss
- ► Consuming a medicine or poison
- ► Allergic reaction
- ► Extreme temperatures
- ► Fatigue
- ► Illness
- ► Stress
- ► Not eating
- ► Standing still for long periods
- ► A breath-holding spell

If you were not with your child when she fainted, find out how long your child was unresponsive. Ask about signs and symptoms, such as nausea, vomiting, and sweating. Ask if she was less alert or seemed confused before she fainted.

Contact a medical provider to find out if your child needs medical care.

Head Injuries

What You Should Know

Head injuries often affect the scalp. The scalp has many blood vessels. Even a small cut can cause a lot of bleeding. Most head injuries do not injure the brain. A child with a head injury may have some bruising and swelling of the skin. Sometimes a bump will appear that looks like a "**goose egg**." The size of the bump doesn't relate to how serious the head injury is. Swelling can takes days or weeks to heal.

goose egg Swelling of the skin on the head that is shaped like a large egg.

The main concern with a head injury is bleeding or swelling inside the skull. This can happen even when the skull itself does not look injured. **Internal head injury** refers to damage to the brain. When the head receives a forceful blow, the brain strikes the inside of the skull. This causes some degree of injury. Also, blood and other fluids can build up inside the skull. This places pressure on the brain. Some internal head injuries can be severe enough to cause permanent brain damage or even death.

internal head injury Damage to the brain. When the head receives a forceful blow, the brain strikes the inside of the skull. This causes some degree of injury.

Concussion is a brain injury that can range from mild to severe. Some symptoms are headache, dizziness, and nausea. Other symptoms are confusion, drowsiness, and loss of responsiveness.

concussion A brain injury that can range from mild to severe; some symptoms are headache, dizziness, nausea, confusion, drowsiness, or loss of responsiveness.

A young baby has an opening in the skull, called a **fontanelle**. Often it is called a "soft spot" (**Figure 2**). Although the skull bone has not yet formed, a very tough covering of tissue protects the brain under the soft spot. Injury to the brain in the area of the fontanelle is rare. A soft spot that bulges, however, means that pressure inside the skull is not normal.

fontanelle Opening in the skull of a young baby, often called a soft spot.

What You Should Look For

Look for any of these signs and symptoms of a head injury:

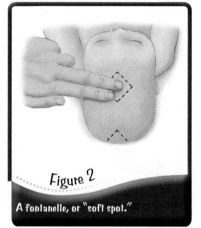

Figure 2

A fontanelle, or "soft spot."

- Bleeding from any part of the head.
- Loss of responsiveness. Appearing stunned for several seconds after a head injury is not the same as being unresponsive. Unresponsiveness can last for just a few seconds or for as long as several days. Crying right after the injury is a good sign.
- Signs of confusion or memory loss. A child should know where she is. She should remember what happened even if she is upset.
- Pale, sweaty appearance.
- Severe headache.
- Nausea or vomiting.
- Blurred vision.
- Unusual sleepiness, listlessness, or tiring easily.
- Irritability, crankiness.
- Pupils that are not equal in size. Check to see if pupils get smaller when exposed to light (**Figure 3**).
- Trouble with walking, speech, or balance.
- Seizure.
- Swelling of a baby's fontanelle.
- Fluid (bloody or clear) dripping from the nose or ear.

Keep Your Child Safe from Motor Vehicle Crashes

Motor vehicle crashes are among the most common causes of head injury in children.

▸ Use a car safety seat for every trip—even short ones.

▸ Select a car safety seat that fits your child's size and age.

▸ Make sure the car safety seat is installed correctly.

▸ Use a booster seat on every trip for children who have outgrown their car safety seats.

See more ways to keep your child safe in and around cars in *Chapter 15: How Do I Keep My Child Safe?* Get more information about selecting, installing, and using car safety seats online at http://www.healthychildren .org/carseatguide.

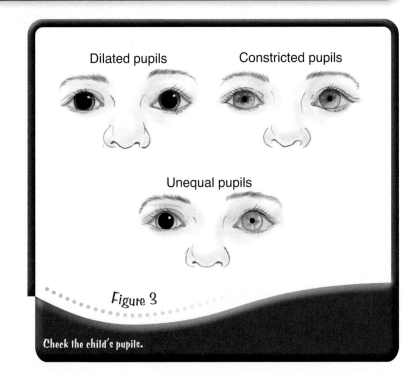

Dilated pupils Constricted pupils

Unequal pupils

Figure 3

Check the child's pupils.

If the child vomits before she is fully responsive, you should roll her entire body and head together to the left side. This is called a **log roll**. This maneuver helps to protect the neck and spine in case of injury. Putting the child on her left side will help reduce vomiting. This position also helps reduce the risk of choking in case the child vomits.

log-roll A maneuver that helps to protect the neck and spine in case of injury.

First Aid Care for Internal (or Suspected Internal) Head Injury

1 If a child is unresponsive, treat the child as if there is a spinal injury.

2 If the child is alert, look at the pupils. Pupils get bigger (dilate) in darkness. They get smaller (constrict) in brighter light. Look to see if the pupils are round and equal to one another. The child's pupils should be about the same size as those of other people in the same light.

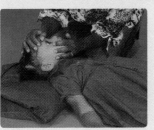

3 Call EMS if your child shows any signs or symptoms of internal head injury listed in "What You Should Look For." Call EMS if the child is unresponsive.

4 If your child is not having any problems, watch her closely for about 6 hours after the injury. Watch for any changes in behavior for the next few days. Talk to your medical provider about the child's injury. Make sure that you understand how to watch for signs and symptoms of a brain injury. Have a plan of action so that you will know what to do in case problems develop.

First Aid for an Open Head Injury

 1 Wear medical gloves if available.

 2 Apply gentle pressure to control any bleeding. Gentle pressure is better than heavy pressure if the skull is fractured.

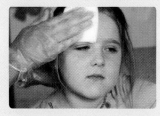

 3 Put a clean bandage on the wound once bleeding has stopped. If the bleeding does not stop with continuous pressure, call EMS.

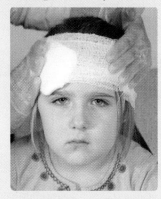

4 Put a cold pack on the injured area for 10 to 15 minutes. (Always protect the skin by wrapping ice or a cold pack in a thin cloth. Direct contact of extreme cold on the skin can cause tissue damage.)

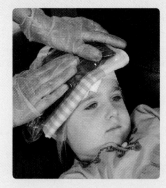

Sleeping After a Head Injury

▶ Let the child sleep if there are no other signs or symptoms of internal head injury and it is a normal bedtime or naptime.

▶ If the child is acting normally before the regular bedtime or naptime, let the child sleep for up to 2 hours without waking her up. After 2 hours of sleeping, wake the child. Check to see if she wakes up as easily as usual. Get medical care if your child is not acting normally.

▶ Note that sleep does not make head injury worse. The concern is that you can't watch a sleeping child for changes in behavior or level of responsiveness.

Diabetic Emergencies

What You Should Know

Low or high blood sugar in a child with diabetes can cause loss of responsiveness. All of the cells in our body depend upon sugar in our blood as the main source of energy. This sugar comes from the foods that we eat. Certain organs in our body also make and store sugar. When the body is working properly, it automatically regulates the amount of sugar in the blood. When there is too much sugar in the blood, the body makes insulin, which lowers blood sugar. When blood sugar levels are too low, the body cuts back on the amount of insulin that it is making and lets the blood sugar levels rise.

Diabetes is a condition in which the body cannot regulate the sugars in the bloodstream. Some children with diabetes must take insulin, either by injection or through an insulin pump. Other children take prescription medicine or have special diets to help manage their diabetes.

diabetes A condition in which the body cannot regulate the sugars in the bloodstream.

When blood sugar levels in the body are lower than normal, a child has **hypoglycemia**. Signs of hypoglycemia in a healthy child are usually mild, such as irritability. In a child with diabetes, hypoglycemia can lead to loss of responsiveness if not treated quickly.

hypoglycemia Blood sugar levels in the body that are lower than normal.

A diabetic child can get hypoglycemia if he doesn't eat enough or doesn't eat at the right time. He can get hypoglycemia if he takes too much insulin. Blood sugar levels may drop because of exercise, being overheated, or illness.

hyperglycemia Blood sugar levels in the body that are higher than normal.

A diabetic child may have too much sugar in the body. This is called **hyperglycemia**. It is the opposite of hypoglycemia. This condition may be caused by too little insulin, illness, or stress. It may be caused by overeating, inactivity, or a combination of all of these factors. See **Table 1** for signs of hypoglycemia and hyperglycemia.

What You Should Look For

Table 1 Hypoglycemia and Hyperglycemia

Signs of Hypoglycemia	Signs of Hyperglycemia
Irritability	Extreme thirst
Paleness	Very frequent urination
Drowsiness	Drowsiness
Confusion	Fruit smell on child's breath
Trembling	Fast breathing
Excessive sweating	Warm, dry skin
Poor coordination	Vomiting
Slurred speech	Eventual loss of responsiveness
Staggering	
Eventual loss of responsiveness	

Hypoglycemia

 If you know your child is diabetic and you have a blood sugar monitor, you should check your child's blood sugar level.

 Give sugar for hypoglycemia. One treatment is to put a teaspoon of granulated sugar on or under the child's tongue. Another treatment is to have the child eat or drink some food containing sugar, such as fruit juice or soda. Don't give diet soda because it doesn't contain sugar.

Hypoglycemia

 If you know your child is diabetic and you have a blood sugar monitor, you should check your child's blood sugar level.

 Give sugar for hypoglycemia. One treatment is to put a teaspoon of granulated sugar on or under the child's tongue. Another treatment is to have the child eat or drink some food containing sugar, such as fruit juice or soda. Don't give diet soda because it doesn't contain sugar.

 If the child does not begin to act normally, call EMS. While waiting for EMS to arrive, give more sugar.

Hyperglycemia

 Call EMS for hyperglycemia.

Not Sure if Child Has Hypoglycemia or Hyperglycemia

 If you are not sure if the child has hypoglycemia or hyperglycemia, give sugar. See if the symptoms improve. Always call EMS if symptoms are severe or if the child becomes unresponsive.

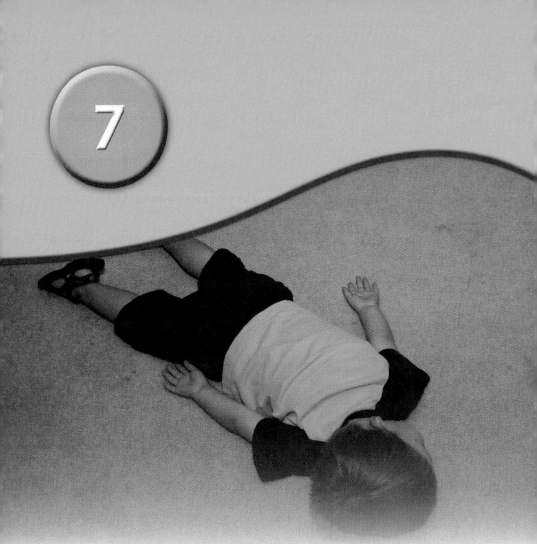

7

Convulsions and Seizures

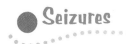 Seizures

Introduction

seizures Medical conditions caused by a disturbance in the electrical impulses of the brain. Seizures can be either convulsive or nonconvulsive.

Seizures are caused by a disturbance in the electrical impulses of the brain. These disturbances cause different responses. Responses range from very mild to more severe. An example of a mild response is a few

78

minutes of blank staring. An example of a more severe response is loss of responsiveness and convulsions.

A seizure can be convulsive or nonconvulsive. Symptoms of a **convulsive seizure** are involuntary muscle contractions and body movement. Symptoms of a **nonconvulsive seizure** are confusion and loss of awareness.

convulsive seizures Involuntary muscle contractions and body movement.

nonconvulsive seizures Seizures with symptoms of confusion and loss of awareness.

What You Should Know

A variety of conditions can cause a seizure. Some of these are an inherited disorder, high fever, or head injury. Serious illness and poisoning are other conditions. If your child has a seizure for the first time, call EMS right away.

Sometimes a specific cause of the seizure can be found, such as a fever. More commonly, the cause is not known. Even without knowing the exact cause, a medical provider can usually treat the child. Medicine can control the seizures or reduce their frequency.

There are different types of seizures. One type is the **generalized seizure with tonic-clonic movement**: rhythmic stiffening and jerking of the trunk and extremities. A child who is having a grand mal seizure will become unresponsive for several seconds. Then he will have violent muscle contractions. Some older children can tell when they are about to have this type of seizure. They recognize a brief feeling that comes on just before the seizure begins. This internal warning is known as an **aura**. It can be a noise, visual change, funny taste, numbness, or other feeling. Some children do not experience an aura. These children don't know when a seizure is about to start.

generalized seizure with tonic-clonic movement A child who is having a grand mal seizure will become unresponsive for several seconds. Then he will have rhythmic stiffening and jerking of trunk and extremities.

aura A feeling that a grand mal seizure is about to begin.

Another type is an **absence seizure**. It only lasts a few seconds. These are characterized by a brief loss of responsiveness or consciousness. The child will suddenly stare off into space for a few seconds and then become responsive again.

absence seizures Seizures with a brief loss of responsiveness. The child will suddenly stare off into space for a few seconds and then become responsive again.

A **febrile seizure** is a seizure caused by a rapid rise in body temperature. The body temperature does not have to be very high, but the rate of change in body temperature is fast. In a number of children, a rapid rise in fever can cause a seizure. A febrile seizure is not related to a lifelong seizure disorder. This type of seizure usually has no effect on the child's nervous system, development, or brain function. Febrile seizures occur most often between 6 months and 6 years of age. A child who has had a febrile seizure is more likely to have another one than a child who has never had one. Febrile seizures usually stop in a few minutes without any special care. A seizure that lasts more than 15 minutes is probably not a febrile seizure. Call EMS if your child has a seizure lasting more than 15 minutes. A child who has a febrile seizure for the first time should be seen by a medical provider as soon as possible. Ask your medical provider for instructions on what to do in case your child has another seizure.

What You Should Look For

The signs and symptoms of seizure include one or more of the following:

- Loss of responsiveness
- Breathing that stops briefly
- Stiff body with jerking and shaking movements of the entire body
- Neck and back arching
- Eyes rolling back
- Increased saliva production, causing drooling or foaming at the mouth
- Loss of control of bladder or bowels

What You Should Do

For any medical situation, follow the Six Steps of Pediatric First Aid. If your child has a seizure, give first aid care. Based on the instructions in "What You Should Do," you will know if you need to call EMS or get medical care.

The Six Steps of Pediatric First Aid

1 **Evaluate the Situation**

Take a few seconds to look around. Evaluate the situation. Make sure the surroundings are safe. Find out who is involved and what happened.

▼

2 **Look and Listen for Signs of an Emergency**

Look and listen for signs that your child's condition is serious or life threatening. Notice the ABCs (Appearance, Breathing, and Circulation). Always call emergency medical services (EMS) for life-threatening conditions. To call EMS, dial 911.

▼

3 **Check for Problems**

Take a closer look and check your child for problems. Use the "What You Should Look For" sections to guide you. Figure out what is wrong, how serious it is, and what you should do next.

▼

4 **Act**

Based on what is wrong, take action. Read the "What You Should Do" sections to be prepared. For a simple injury, you may only need to give first aid. For a serious condition, you may need to call EMS and give care until help arrives.

▼

5 **Follow Up**

Be sure to follow up. Give any care or treatment that your child might need after the event.

▼

6 **Prevent**

Take steps to prevent the illness or injury from happening again, if possible. Prevention is as important as first aid in caring for your child.

First Aid Care for Convulsive Seizures

 Position the child on his left side to let saliva drain and to keep the tongue from blocking the airway. This position also helps reduce the risk of choking in case the child vomits.

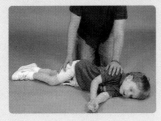

 Loosen any tight clothing.

3 Call EMS and give CPR if the child is blue or is not breathing.

4 Never put anything into the child's mouth.

5 Move toys and furniture out of the way.

6 Slide the palm of your hand under the child's head to protect the head from injury. Also, you can protect the child's head with a towel, blanket, or clothing.

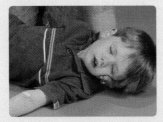

 Note the time the seizure begins and ends. Observe the body parts affected. A seizure might seem to last longer than it actually does, especially if you are frightened. It is important to tell your child's medical provider what happened just before, during, and after the seizure.

 Call EMS if your child has not had a seizure before. If your child has had a seizure before, follow your medical provider's instructions.

Let your child rest while lying on his side (the recovery position) after the seizure. Recovery from a seizure is usually slow. He will sleep or be drowsy for a while. Some children will be overactive after a seizure.

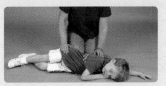

 If your child has a fever and you have instructions from your medical provider, give a fever-reducing medicine. Examples of fever-reducing medicines are acetaminophen or ibuprofen. Give this medicine when your child can swallow it safely.

 Follow the care plan for seizures from your medical provider.

First Aid Care for Nonconvulsive Seizures

 Time the seizure. Watch the body parts affected if movements occur.

 Make sure your child is in a place where he will not be hurt if he moves during the seizure.

3 Let the child rest if needed.

4 Follow the care plan for seizures from your medical provider.

First Aid TIP

▶ Don't force anything between your child's teeth.
▶ Don't restrain your child's movements.
▶ Protect your child from his environment.
▶ Don't give your child anything to eat or drink until he is fully alert.

Allergic Reactions

allergy An abnormal reaction of the body's immune system to a certain substance.

allergen A substance that causes an allergic reaction. Some common allergens are molds, dust, animal dander, pollen, foods, and medicines. Cleaning products and other chemicals are also common allergens. The body perceives allergens as dangerous.

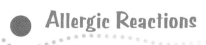

Allergic Reactions

Introduction

An **allergy** is an abnormal reaction of the body's immune system to a certain substance. The substance that causes this reaction is called an **allergen**. Some common allergens are molds, dust, animal dander, pollen, foods, and medicine. Cleaning products and other chemicals are also common allergens. The body perceives allergens as dangerous. Contact with an allergen will trigger an allergic reaction. **Allergic reactions** can cause hives and tissue swelling (**Figure 1**). Some common symptoms are runny nose, watery eyes, swollen lips, and itchy throat. Other common symptoms are coughing, trouble breathing, wheezing, and rash. Although it is rare, allergies can cause anaphylaxis. **Anaphylaxis** is a life-threatening type of allergic reaction that can cause the airway to swell and blood pressure to fall.

allergic reaction The body's response to an allergen, often as hives or tissue swelling.

anaphylaxis A life-threatening type of allergic reaction that can cause the airway to swell.

If you know that your child has allergies, be prepared to act quickly in case of an allergic reaction. Sometimes your medical provider will prescribe an antihistamine or asthma medicine to treat an allergic reaction. If your child is at risk for anaphylactic reaction, your medical provider will prescribe an epinephrine auto-injector. **Epinephrine** is a hormone that stops the airway from swelling. Epinephrine in an auto-injector is often marketed as Epi-Pen and Epi-Pen, Jr (**Figure 2**). You should be trained by your medical provider on how to use the auto-injector.

epinephrine A hormone that stops the effects of anaphylaxis.

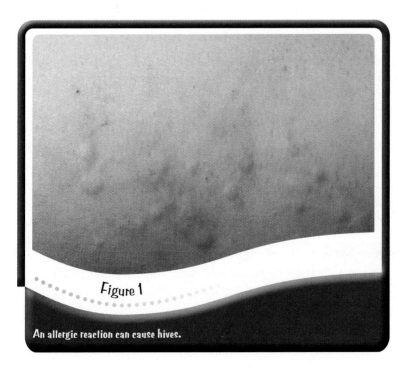

Figure 1

An allergic reaction can cause hives.

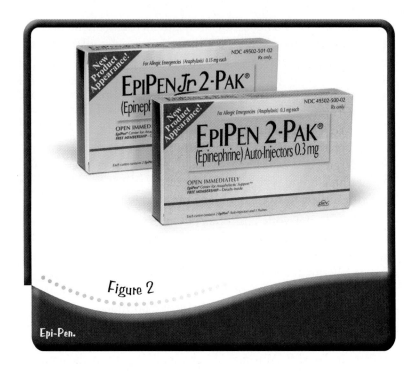

Figure 2

Epi-Pen.

What You Should Know

Anaphylaxis is a severe allergic reaction. It is a type of shock that can be fatal if not reversed within minutes. Anaphylaxis comes on suddenly, usually within seconds or minutes after a child comes in contact with the allergen. Anaphylaxis can cause airway swelling that cuts off the child's ability to breathe. If epinephrine is not available, death can occur within minutes.

Anaphylaxis can be unexpected. You may not know that your child has an extreme allergy to a substance that is harmless to most people. Anaphylaxis is a rare type of allergic reaction. It is more likely to be caused by insect stings or food allergies. Environmental allergens, such as molds, dust, animal dander, and pollen, do not usually cause anaphylaxis.

Anaphylaxis occurs more often in a child who has been exposed at least once, and usually multiple times, to one of the following:

- Insect stings from bees, wasps, hornets, yellow jackets, or ants
- A medicine
- A food, such as shellfish, nuts, eggs, or milk

Usually, anaphylaxis is not the first type of allergic reaction a child will have when exposed to one of these substances. However, the exposures that trigger an allergic reaction might not be obvious. A child might eat a prepared food without knowing that it contains an allergic ingredient.

Children who have had an extreme allergic reaction to a specific allergen should have an epinephrine auto-injector. Store the auto-injector at room temperature with the first aid supplies. An auto-injector is not a routine item in first aid kits; it is a prescription drug intended only for the child with allergies in an emergency. The auto-injector is an easy-to-use device that gives the correct dose of epinephrine. See *Chapter 9: Bites and Stings* for instructions on using an epinephrine auto-injector for severe allergic reactions. The auto-injector must always be close at hand wherever your child goes. This means that the auto-injector should go out to the playground or to sports events with the first aid supplies. It should go on field trips and on visits to friends and relatives.

Children allergic to certain foods can usually be protected from exposure. Don't allow a child with allergies to share food. Some child care facilities and schools restrict the types of foods that children can bring. They try to educate parents and caregivers about foods that contain ingredients that may be harmful to someone with allergies. It is hard, however, to educate everyone who may prepare foods for a child.

Separating a child with allergies from her classmates during snack and meal times may be correct in severe cases, but it can make a child feel isolated. Work with your child's school or facility to make the best of the situation. If other children are eating foods that might pose a hazard, then your child should be separated. Try to arrange for her to be part of a small supervised group instead of putting her in a separate place all alone.

Did You Know?

An allergy can develop at any time in life, no matter how often a person has been exposed to the substance in the past.

Did You Know?

Shock is a condition that can be caused by many factors. Some factors that cause shock are allergic reaction, dehydration, loss of blood, and infection. The general treatment for shock is to call EMS and keep the child warm and calm. The child should lie down with his feet slightly raised, unless you suspect a spinal injury. Cover the child with a blanket to keep him warm. If he is bleeding, try to control any more loss of blood. If the shock is related to an allergy and an epinephrine auto-injector is available, use it.

Did You Know?

Common food allergies include:

▶ Chocolate
▶ Eggs
▶ Milk
▶ Nuts
▶ Peanuts
▶ Shellfish
▶ Soybeans
▶ Wheat

Did You Know?

In some locations, EMS providers can give epinephrine shots. In others, they cannot. Then the child must wait until reaching the emergency room unless you have your own prescription epinephrine auto-injector. Find out if your local EMS can give epinephrine and plan accordingly.

Did You Know?

People with allergies should avoid substances that cause allergic symptoms as much as possible. Read all food labels carefully when a child has food allergies. For example, whey and casein are milk products that are added to many types of crackers. Check with The Food Allergy & Anaphylaxis Network for tips on hidden ingredients in foods. They also have training kits to teach parents and caregivers about handling food allergies. Go online to http://www.foodallergy.org or call 1-800-929-4040.

Be aware that some children with allergies are very sensitive. They can have an allergic response if they even touch a surface that has been touched by someone eating a food that contains the allergen. The only way to protect such children is to ban the food from the environment of that child altogether.

What You Should Look For

- Swelling of the face, lips, and throat
- Wheezing/shortness of breath
- Tightness in the chest
- Dizziness
- Blue/gray color around lips
- Nausea and vomiting
- Drooling
- Itchy skin, hives, or other rashes appearing quickly

What You Should Do

For any emergency situation, follow the Six Steps of Pediatric First Aid. If your child is having a severe allergic reaction, call EMS. Give first aid care as described in "What You Should Do."

The Six Steps of Pediatric First Aid

 1 **Evaluate the Situation**

Take a few seconds to look around. Evaluate the situation. Make sure the surroundings are safe. Find out who is involved and what happened.

▼

2 **Look and Listen for Signs of an Emergency**

Look and listen for signs that your child's condition is serious or life threatening. Notice the ABCs (Appearance, Breathing, and Circulation). Always call emergency medical services (EMS) for life-threatening conditions. To call EMS, dial 911.

▼

3 **Check for Problems**

Take a closer look and check your child for problems. Use the "What You Should Look For" sections to guide you. Figure out what is wrong, how serious it is, and what you should do next.

▼

 4 **Act**

Based on what is wrong, take action. Read the "What You Should Do" sections to be prepared. For a simple injury, you may only need to give first aid. For a serious condition, you may need to call EMS and give care until help arrives.

▼

5 **Follow Up**

Be sure to follow up. Give any care or treatment that your child might need after the event.

▼

6 **Prevent**

Take steps to prevent the illness or injury from happening again, if possible. Prevention is as important as first aid in caring for your child.

First Aid Care for Anaphylaxis

 Place an unresponsive child on his left side. Check for breathing and call EMS. If the child is not breathing, give CPR.

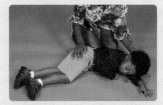

 Place a responsive child who is having trouble breathing in a sitting position to make breathing easier. Call EMS.

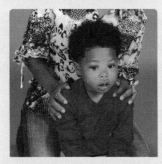

 If a child has an epinephrine auto-injector, give it right away. Follow the manufacturer's instructions on how to use it. A second injection may be needed if EMS does not arrive within 15 minutes of the first injection. If your child does not have an auto-injector, watch him closely for problems with breathing. Give an antihistamine or asthma medicine if prescribed by your medical provider.

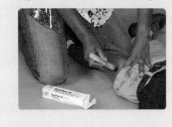

First Aid TIP

How to Use an Epinephrine Auto-Injector for a Severe Allergic Reaction

▶ Call EMS.

▶ Don't remove the safety cap until you are ready to use the medicine.

▶ Never put your fingers over the black ejection tip while removing the gray safety cap or after you have given the medicine.

▶ Do not use the auto-injector if:

   — It is not prescribed for your child.

   — It is discolored (yellow versus clear).

   — There are particles in it.

   — It is older than the expiration date printed on the side of the box.

▶ Hold the auto-injector in your hand and make a fist around it. Remove the auto-injector's safety cap.

▶ Place the black tip of the injector directly against the child's outer thigh (you can inject through clothing). Inject the medicine into the fleshy outer portion of the thigh. Do not inject the medicine into a vein or the buttocks.

▶ With a quick motion, push the auto-injector firmly against the thigh. Hold it in place until all the medicine is injected—usually no more than 10 seconds.

▶ Remove the injector and put it back into its safety tube. Give it to the EMS providers when they arrive.

▶ Massage the area after the injection.

Did You Know?

▶ More than one dose of epinephrine may be needed to reverse anaphylaxis.

▶ A second dose can be given after 15 minutes if needed.

▶ Epinephrine can cause a fast heart rate, pale skin, and nausea.

9

Bites and Stings

● Bites and Stings

Introduction

Animal and human bites are common sources of injury to young children. Many animals and insects that can cause injury are specific to certain parts of the country. For instance, ticks and mosquitoes are common in wet climates; scorpions are found in dry desert areas.

You should know how to give first aid care for common types of bites or stings in your area. The **Poison Help hotline** can tell you about local risks and what to do if your child gets a bite or sting. If you have an emergency from a poisonous bite or sting, call 1-800-222-1222. For more information, go to the American Association of Poison Control Centers website at www.aapcc.org.

Most of the time, bites and stings are more of a nuisance than a serious health problem. Some bites and stings, however, can be more serious and require urgent medical care. Be prepared to give first aid to relieve your child's pain and discomfort. Know what to look for and how to decide if your child needs medical care right away.

Animal and Human Bites

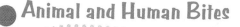

What You Should Know

About 90% of animal bites in the United States each year are from dogs. Cats are less likely to bite than dogs. Cat bite wounds, however, are more likely to become infected and cause a life-threatening

Did You Know?

Keep Your Children Safe from Dog Bites by Teaching Them How to Behave Around Dogs

▶ Don't go near an unfamiliar dog.

▶ Don't run from a dog or scream.

▶ Don't move (e.g., "be still like a tree") when approached by an unfamiliar dog.

▶ If knocked over by a dog, roll into a ball, and lie still (e.g., "be still like a log").

▶ Don't play with a dog unless supervised by an adult.

▶ Report a stray dog or a dog that is acting funny to an adult.

▶ Don't look directly into a dog's eyes.

▶ Don't disturb a dog that is sleeping, eating, or caring for puppies.

▶ Don't pet a dog without letting it see and sniff you first.

▶ If a dog bites you, report it to an adult right away.

Source: Modified from CDC, Injury Prevention & Control: Home and Recreational Safety, Dog Bite Prevention [http://www.cdc.gov/homeandrecreationalsafety/dog-bites/biteprevention.html]. Accessed July 23, 2010.

situation. Other animals that bite are ferrets and monkeys. Wild animals that have been known to bite humans are squirrels, chipmunks, foxes, and raccoons. The teeth of an animal carry many bacteria. Any animal bite that breaks the skin can become infected. Some animals may spread disease when they bite.

rabies A life-threatening viral disease in warm-blooded mammals that is most often transferred through bites.

The most dangerous infection that can develop after an animal bite is rabies. **Rabies** is a viral disease. Any warm-blooded animal can carry rabies, but it is found mostly in wild animals. Commonly infected animals are raccoons, bats, foxes, and coyotes. A bite from a stray cat or dog is a concern because stray animals are probably not immunized (**Figure 1**). Caged animals, such as hamsters, gerbils, and guinea pigs, typically do not carry rabies.

A child can get rabies from the bite of an animal that is infected. Rabies affects the brain and the nervous system. Once symptoms develop, the disease is fatal. If your child gets a bite or scratch from a wild animal, get medical care right away. Your child must be checked for rabies. Your child should get medical care if she is bitten or scratched by any pet that has not been immunized. Try to confirm the pet's rabies vaccine status from the pet's owner. Never try to capture or restrain the animal.

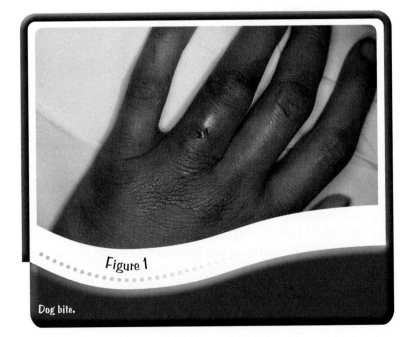

Figure 1

Dog bite.

Human bites are common in groups of toddlers. Sometimes a child bites because she is angry or frustrated. Many of these bites are minor and do not break the skin. They cause more of an emotional upset than a physical injury. Any bite that breaks the skin, whether animal or human, can cause a serious infection.

What You Should Look For

- Surface breaks on the skin with little or no bleeding
- Puncture-type wounds
- Cuts
- Crushing injuries
- Torn tissues in the area of the bite

What You Should Do

For any medical situation, follow the Six Steps of Pediatric First Aid. If your child gets a bite or sting, give first aid care. Based on the type of bite or sting, you will be able to decide if you need to call EMS or get medical care.

The Six Steps of Pediatric First Aid

1 Evaluate the Situation

Take a few seconds to look around. Evaluate the situation. Make sure the surroundings are safe. Find out who is involved and what happened.

▼

2 Look and Listen for Signs of an Emergency

Look and listen for signs that your child's condition is serious or life threatening. Notice the ABCs (Appearance, Breathing, and Circulation). Always call emergency medical services (EMS) for life-threatening conditions. To call EMS, dial 911.

▼

3 Check for Problems

Take a closer look and check your child for problems. Use the "What You Should Look For" sections to guide you. Figure out what is wrong, how serious it is, and what you should do next.

▼

4 **Act**

Based on what is wrong, take action. Read the "What You Should Do" sections to be prepared. For a simple injury, you may only need to give first aid. For a serious condition, you may need to call EMS and give care until help arrives.

▼

5 **Follow Up**

Be sure to follow up. Give any care or treatment that your child might need after the event.

▼

6 **Prevent**

Take steps to prevent the illness or injury from happening again, if possible. Prevention is as important as first aid in caring for your child.

First Aid Care for Bites from Dogs, Cats, Other Animals, and Humans

1 Remove the child and others from area. Call EMS if the bite caused serious injury or if you can't control bleeding. Call EMS, even if the wound seems minor, for any of the following:

- ► A bite from a skunk, raccoon, bat, fox, coyote, or other wild animal.
- ► A bite from any animal that is acting strangely. The strange behavior may be a sign of rabies.
- ► A bite from any animal that is not known to be up-to-date with a rabies vaccine.

2 Care for any wound or bruised area. Wash any area where the skin is broken with soap and rinse with water. This will help reduce the risk of infection. If the skin is not broken, clean the area with soap and water. Cover the area with a cloth and apply ice or a cold pack to reduce pain and swelling. Always protect the skin by wrapping ice or a cold pack in a thin cloth. Direct contact of extreme cold on the skin can cause tissue damage.

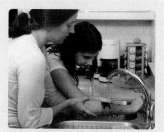

3 If your child was bitten by a dog or cat, contact the animal's owner. You need to verify that the animal's rabies vaccine is up-to-date. Check with your local health department or animal control officer to find out what to do with the animal. The animal may need to be confined and watched for signs of rabies. A veterinarian should evaluate the animal.

Insect Bites and Stings

What You Should Know

Children are naturally curious and want to explore. As a result, they can come in contact with bees, wasps, yellow jackets, hornets, and fire ants (**Figure 2A–C**). Children may attract insects from leftover food on their clothes or hands. In most cases, a child who is stung by an insect does not need medical care. A severe allergic reaction to an insect sting, however, can happen quickly without warning. This type of severe allergic reaction is called anaphylaxis. It may be life threatening. See *Chapter 8: Allergic Reactions* to learn more.

Many insects bite or sting. Symptoms of an insect bite or sting are caused from venom that is injected into the skin. **Venom** is a poisonous fluid that insects make. Venom can cause both irritation and an allergic reaction. The venom or stinger may also cause infection. Insects are not usually aggressive. They attack only when threatened or when their hives or nests are disturbed. Then they sting, sometimes in swarms. A child may threaten a stinging insect by running into it or playing near its hive.

venom A poisonous fluid that insects and snakes make.

97

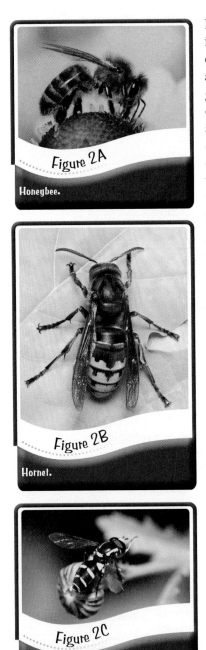

Figure 2A

Honeybee.

Figure 2B

Hornet.

Figure 2C

Wasp.

Normal reactions to an insect sting are pain, itching, and swelling. These disappear in a day or so. Mild allergic reactions are hives and swelling. For someone with severe allergies, hives and swelling may be symptoms of a severe reaction or anaphylaxis. Severe allergic reactions vary in intensity. They can occur within minutes to several hours after contact with the insect venom. Medical providers prescribe the epinephrine auto-injector for children at risk for anaphylaxis.

Biting insects are mosquitoes, gnats, chiggers, and some types of flies. In many areas of the country, these insects can spread diseases that are specific to that area. The insects inject the germs that cause the disease along with their saliva when they puncture the skin. Usually, insect bites itch and are annoying for a few days but cause no other problems.

Mosquitoes and gnats are most active around dawn and dusk. They are also active when it is humid. Chiggers are microscopic mites. They attach to skin with tiny claws and feed on liquids inside human skin cells. They are most likely to attach in places where clothing is tighter. Examples are tops of socks and under the elastic band of underwear.

Although many insects can bite, most avoid contact with people. Some insects are attractive to children, even though they would rather be left alone. For example, children love to handle caterpillars. Many caterpillars can cause a rash.

Local health authorities have information about disease risks from biting insects in your area. Ask the local health department or your medical provider about what to watch for and safe ways to reduce the risk of insect bites in children.

What You Should Look For

- Painful or itchy area at the site of the sting or bite
- Redness and swelling of the area
- Child feels or acts sick
- Signs of an allergic reaction, such as:
    - Hives, spreading rash, large amount of swelling
    - Trouble breathing
    - Dry, hacking cough, wheezing, or tightness in nose, throat, or chest
    - Itchy eyes
    - Swelling of lips, eyes, or throat
    - Weakness or dizziness
    - Fast heartbeat
    - Nausea/vomiting

First Aid Care for Mild to Moderate Reactions to Insect Stings and Bites

 Move the child to a safe area to avoid more stings or bites.

Remove any part of the stinging or biting insect that's left. Look for and quickly remove any stinger by scraping it with a credit card or fingernail. If your child has touched a caterpillar that left any of its spines on the skin, remove the spines with the sticky side of tape.

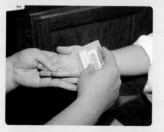

 Wash the area with soap and rinse with water.

First Aid Care for Mild to
Moderate Reactions to Insect
Stings and Bites (continued)

 Cover the area with a cloth and apply ice or a cold pack to reduce pain and swelling. Always protect the skin by wrapping ice or a cold pack in a thin cloth. Direct contact of extreme cold on the skin can cause tissue damage.

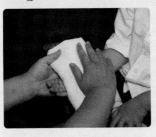

 Keep the area elevated above the heart.

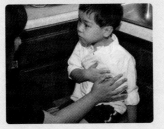

 If your medical provider has prescribed an antihistamine or other medicine for insect stings or bites, give the medicine right away. If you gave a prescribed auto-injector, call EMS right away.

Watch your child for any other reactions to the sting or bite. Also watch for reactions to the medicine.

Did You Know?

Honeybees leave a sack attached to their stinger in the skin. The sack continues to pump venom into the bite site for a few seconds after the sting. Getting it out right away can reduce the amount of venom that irritates the tissues. Yellow jackets and some wasps also leave a stinger in the skin. Stingers carry many bacteria. Taking the stinger out reduces the risk of infection.

How to Protect Your Child from Insect Stings

▶ Check for nests in areas where children play. Nests can be found in old tree stumps, around rotting wood, and in holes in the ground. Check in auto tires that are part of a playground. Look around trash cans.

▶ Have insect nests removed by a professional exterminator.

▶ Don't allow children who are allergic to insects to play outside alone when stinging insects are active. Even a dead insect can sting if a child steps on it or picks it up.

▶ Wear shoes. Avoid wearing sandals or going barefoot.

▶ Avoid wearing bright colors and floral patterns. These can attract insects. Wear white, green, tan, and khaki. These colors are not as attractive to insects.

▶ When eating outdoors, avoid foods that attract insects. Some examples are tuna, peanut butter and jelly sandwiches, and watermelon. Sweetened drinks, frozen sweet treats, and ice cream also attract insects.

▶ Stay away from garbage cans and dumpsters.

▶ If an insect is near, do not swat at it or run. These actions can trigger an attack. Walk away slowly. If you have disturbed a nest and the insects swarm around you, curl up as tightly as you can to reduce exposed skin. Keep your face down and cover your head with your arms.

▶ A child who is allergic to insects should wear a medical alert necklace or bracelet.

Tick Bites

What You Should Know

A tick is a tiny brown mite that attaches itself to the skin of an animal or human to suck blood (**Figures 3** and **4**). Ticks do not fly or jump; they attach themselves to an animal or human who brushes up against them. Diseases carried by ticks are Lyme disease, Rocky Mountain spotted fever, and Colorado tick fever. Other diseases are tick paralysis and tularemia (can be caused by ticks or rabbits). Many tick bites do not cause disease.

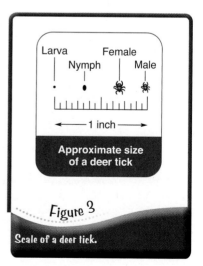

Larva   Female
Nymph   Male

◀— 1 inch —▶

Approximate size of a deer tick

Figure 3

Scale of a deer tick.

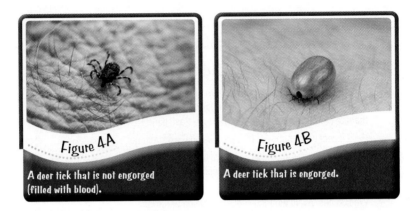

Figure 4A

A deer tick that is not engorged (filled with blood).

Figure 4B

A deer tick that is engorged.

Ticks must feed on blood to survive. It is during these feedings that disease can be spread to humans. As the tick feeds, it deposits the waste from its gut into the wound where it is feeding. Infection is less likely to occur if the tick is removed before it has time to feed and fill with blood. The risk of being bitten by an infected tick is greatest in the summer months, especially in May and June. In some areas, ticks can be a year-round threat. The risk of being bitten depends upon your location. It also depends upon how much time your child spends outdoors in wooded or tall grassy areas. Some methods are better than others to prevent tick bites. Local health authorities have information about the risk of tick-borne disease and how to reduce the risk of tick bites.

What You Should Look For

An embedded tick or a bump on the skin that is new.

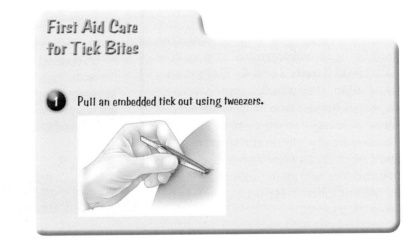

First Aid Care for Tick Bites

1. Pull an embedded tick out using tweezers.

Grasp the tick as close to the skin as possible. Lift it in the same direction as it entered the skin. Pull with enough force to "tent" the skin surface. Hold it in that position until the tick lets go. This may take several seconds. Don't twist or jerk the tick. Twisting or jerking may cause some of the tick to be left in the wound made by the tick's bite. Don't grab a tick at the rear of its body. The body may rupture. Then the infectious contents could enter the wound.

 Wash the bite area with soap and rinse with water.

4 Watch the area of the tick bite for several weeks to see if a rash appears. If your child gets a rash or becomes sick, get medical care.

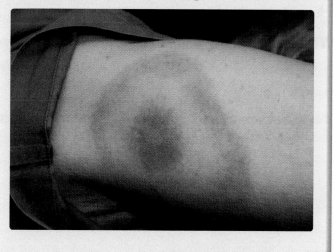

First Aid TIP

Don't use any of the following ineffective methods of tick removal:

▶ Petroleum jelly
▶ Fingernail polish
▶ Rubbing alcohol
▶ Kerosene or gasoline
▶ A match head that is blown out but is still hot

What You Should Know

The United States has 120 species of snakes. Only 20 are poisonous. Almost every state has at least one species of poisonous snake (**Figure 5**). The only states that don't are Maine, Hawaii, and Alaska. In some areas, snakes may invade playgrounds after heavy rains.

Flooding of snake burrows makes snakes look for drier ground. All snakes can bite, but snakes generally try to avoid people when they can. Although a snakebite from a poisonous snake is a serious injury, deaths from poisonous snakes are unusual. Some poisonous snakes are rattlesnakes, copperheads, coral snakes, and cottonmouth water moccasins (**Figure 6A–D**).

What You Should Look For

- Two small puncture wounds about one-half inch apart (sometimes there may be only one fang mark)

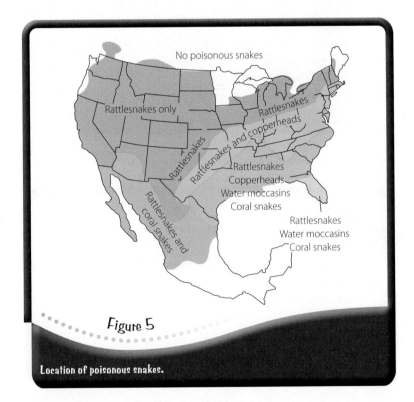

Figure 5

Location of poisonous snakes.

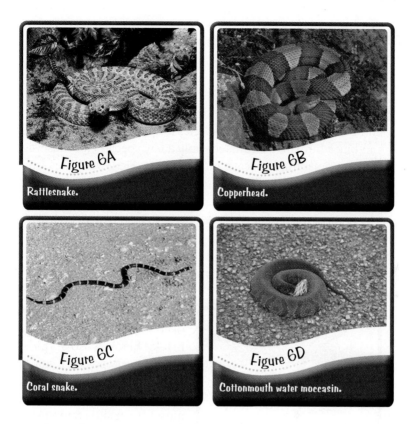

Figure 6A

Rattlesnake.

Figure 6B

Copperhead.

Figure 6C

Coral snake.

Figure 6D

Cottonmouth water moccasin.

- Severe burning pain at the bite site
- Rapid swelling
- Discoloration (turns blue or red) or blood-filled blisters (may develop within 6 to 10 hours)
- In severe cases, nausea, vomiting, sweating, trouble breathing, and weakness

First Aid Care for Snakebites

 Get child and others away from the snake.

2 Keep the child quiet and the body part still to slow the spread of venom. The bitten arm or leg should be kept at or lower than the child's heart. This will help keep the venom from spreading in the body.

3 Call EMS and the Poison Help hotline (1-800-222-1222).

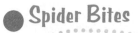

Spider Bites

What You Should Know

Most spiders are poisonous. They use their poison to paralyze and kill their prey. About 60 species of spiders in North America can bite a human. Fortunately, only a few species can cause significant poisonings. Death rarely occurs. However, bites from the black widow and brown recluse spiders have been known to cause death.

The body of the female black widow is shaped like an hourglass. She is a dark color with red or yellow on the abdomen (**Figure 7**). Black widow spiders are found in all 48 contiguous states. Only the female is dangerous. The male is too small to bite through human skin.

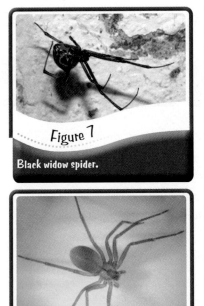

Figure 7

Black widow spider.

Brown recluse spider.

Figure 8

The bite itself often goes unnoticed or may be felt as a pinprick. Black widow spider venom is very potent. It attacks the muscles in humans. Symptoms are often severe muscle pain and cramping.

The brown recluse spider is also known as the fiddle-back or violin spider (**Figure 8**). A violin-shaped marking on the back helps to identify it. Both the male and female are dangerous.

It is rare to see the brown recluse spider when it bites because the bite is painless. Most bites happen while the person is sleeping. Reactions to a bite from a brown recluse vary. They range from mild irritation at the bite site to a potentially fatal poisoning.

What You Should Look For

- Tiny fang marks
- Pain
- Pain begins as a dull ache at the bite site
- Pain spreads to the surrounding muscles
- Pain moves to the abdomen, back, chest, and legs
- Blister at the bite site
- Mild swelling and a blue-gray mark at the bite surrounded by lightening of skin color
- Progressive soft tissue damage; the skin becomes dark blue and then black (necrotic)

First Aid TIP

1. Don't use the "cut-and-suck" method to remove venom.
2. Don't use mouth suction. The human mouth is filled with bacteria. This would increase the chance of infection.
3. Don't apply a tight band around an arm or leg. That can cause more harm.
4. Call EMS right away.

First Aid Care for Spider Bites

 If you suspect that your child has been bitten by a brown recluse or black widow spider, call EMS. Wash the bite area with soap and rinse with water.

Cover the area with a cloth and apply ice or a cold pack. This will help relieve pain and delay the effects of the venom. (Always protect the skin by wrapping ice or a cold pack in a thin cloth. Direct contact of extreme cold on the skin can cause tissue damage.)

First Aid Care for Spider Bites
(continued)

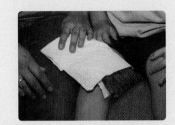

3 Call the Poison Help hotline (1-800-222-1222).

Did You Know?

For black widow spider bites there is an **antidote** that can counteract the effects of the poison. It is usually reserved for young children (younger than 6 years), the elderly (older than 60 years), and those with severe reactions. An antidote for brown recluse and other spiders is not available.

Scorpion Stings

What You Should Know

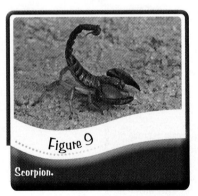

Figure 9

Scorpion.

Scorpions look like miniature lobsters. They have pincers and a long up-curved tail with a poisonous stinger (**Figure 9**). Several species of scorpions live in the southwestern United States, but only the bark scorpion poses a threat to humans. Severe reactions to the sting of the bark scorpion are usually only seen in children. Some of these reactions are paralysis, spasms, or trouble breathing. The bark scorpion is pale tan in color. It is ¾ to 1¼ inches long, not including the tail.

What You Should Look For

- Pain in the area of the sting that gets worse in several minutes. Pain may travel up the limb that was stung.
- Mild swelling.

First Aid Care for Scorpion Stings

1 Call EMS.

2 Wash the sting site with soap and rinse with water.

3 Cover the area with a cloth and apply ice or a cold pack to the sting site to reduce pain. (Always protect the skin by wrapping ice or a cold pack in a thin cloth. Direct contact of extreme cold on the skin can cause tissue damage.)

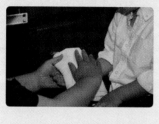

Marine Animal Stings

What You Should Know

Each year, marine animals sting more than one million people. Examples of marine animals are jellyfish and the Portuguese man-of-war. They lie along shallow ocean waters. These animals sting by firing special tentacles called **nematocysts**. Nematocysts contain poison. This is how these animals capture their prey and defend themselves against attack. It is important to identify the animal that stung your child because in many cases care is quite specific.

> **nematocysts** Stinging tentacles fired by marine animals to capture their prey or to defend themselves.

Reactions to being stung vary from mild irritation to severe reactions.

What You Should Look For

- A raised bump or ridge with redness
- Burning pain
- Muscle cramping

First Aid Care for Marine Animal Stings

 Remove the child from the water.

 Rinse the skin with seawater.

Pour vinegar on the affected area until pain is relieved. Unlike fresh water, vinegar will make the nematocysts inactive.

Try to remove the loose tentacles by scraping them off with the edge of a sharp, stiff object, such as a credit card. Don't handle tentacles with bare hands.

10

Poisoning

Poisoning

Introduction

A **poison** is a substance that can cause harm to the body or even death if you eat, drink, touch, or breathe it. Poisons can be solid, such as pills (over-the-counter medications and vitamins), batteries, plants, and

poison A substance that can cause harm to the body or even death if you eat, drink, touch, or breathe it.

berries. Poisons can be liquid, such as antifreeze, lamp oil, and household cleaners. Poisons can be sprays, such as bug spray, weed killer, or furniture polish. Poisons can be invisible and have no smell, such as carbon monoxide. Often exposure to only a tiny amount of a poison can be life threatening. Poisoning is one of the most common causes of injury in children younger than 5 years old.

You can call 1-800-222-1222 to reach the Poison Help hotline, which is staffed by medical professionals. Keep this number posted by each phone in your house (**Figure 1**). The Poison Help hotline gives free advice. It is available 24 hours a day, 7 days a week, 365 days a year. It is a resource not only for parents but also for medical providers, nurses, and pharmacists. The Poison Help hotline staff members have access to the most current information about every poisoning situation. They will tell you what you should do first and if you need to call EMS. Go to their website at http://www.aapcc.org for more information on poisoning and poisoning prevention.

What You Should Know

Many products that you use every day are poisonous. The poisons that are most harmful to children are medicines, cleaning

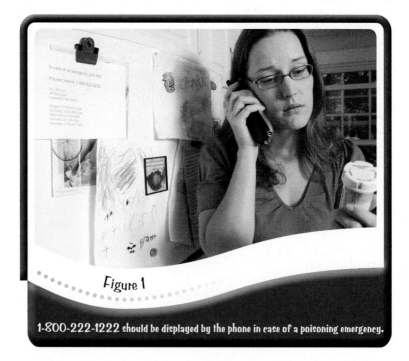

Figure 1

1-800-222-1222 should be displayed by the phone in case of a poisoning emergency.

Here are some poisons frequently found in and around the home. Make sure your child cannot get to them:

Furniture polish	Hair relaxers	Gasoline
Spray cleaners	Perm solutions	Kerosene
Drain opener	Hair-coloring products	Paint thinner
Floor cleaner	Nail polish remover	Lamp oil
Toilet cleaner	Mouthwash	Antifreeze
Oven cleaner	Cosmetics	Windshield washer fluid
Laundry detergents	Perfume	Pesticides
Alcoholic beverages	Nail polish	Roach tablets
Prescription medicines	Deodorant	Rat poison
Over-the-counter medicines	Soap	Rust remover
Cough syrup	Batteries	Bug spray
Vitamins	Cigarettes	Poisonous houseplants
Pet medicines	Lighter fluid	Poisonous outdoor plants

Did You Know?

Child-resistant safety packaging for medicine bottles was developed in the 1970s. There is no such thing as "childproof packaging." Given enough time, a child can figure out how to get the bottle open. This type of packaging does make it harder for the child to open the bottle so that an adult has a better chance of finding the child first.

Did You Know?

One of the leading causes of childhood poisoning is acetaminophen. It is a significant cause of liver damage and even death.

products, pesticides, alcoholic beverages, and petroleum products, such as gasoline. The leading causes of poisoning in children are:

- Cosmetics, such as perfume or nail polish
- Personal care products, such as deodorant and soap
- Medicines, such as pain killers
- Cleaning products, such as laundry detergent and floor cleaners

Poisonings often happen when parents or caregivers are tired or preoccupied. Children can get into poison if left alone for only a minute.

Many poisons look attractive to children—bright containers with big letters; pills in different shapes and colors; blue, pink, and yellow liquids. Young children are curious by nature and love to explore. Taste is the first sense young children use to investigate something new. It doesn't matter if it is a toy, food, chemical, or plant. Most childhood poisonings can be prevented by proper storage of medicines and household products. Keep anything that is poisonous in locked cabinets; on high, secure shelves; or in boxes that children cannot reach. When you are using a poison, be careful to keep it away from your child. If the phone or door-bell rings, take your child with you to answer it. Don't leave your child where he could have access to a poison for even a minute. When you dispose of a poison, make sure your child can't get to the empty container. Sometimes only a small amount of a poison can be very dangerous.

Like many adults, most young children know little about poisonous plants. It is not unusual for a child to want to touch leaves, berries, and flowers. Small children often want to put everything that they touch into their mouths. A child can be poisoned from swallowing a leaf. A child can absorb poisons through the skin by touching a poisonous plant. A child can even be poisoned by breathing fumes from a fire that contains a poisonous plant. To protect your child, learn the names of the plants, trees, and shrubbery around your house and in your neighborhood. Know which ones are poisonous. Don't overlook house plants—many of those are poisonous as well. Teach your child to identify poisonous plants and to stay away from them. If your child swallows any part of a plant, take the child and a sample of the plant to the telephone. Call the Poison Help hotline at 1-800-222-1222. They will tell you what to do next.

A few plants contain oil that can cause a mild to severe rash. The best known are poison ivy, poison oak, and poison sumac (**Figure 2**). All of these are found throughout the United States. A reaction can develop from contact with these plants during any season of the year (**Figure 3**).

A child can come in contact with the oil of the plant *directly* by handling any part of the plant, not just the leaves. A child can come in contact with this oil *indirectly* by touching tools, clothes, pets, or anything else that has been touched by the plant. Smoke from a fire containing the burning plant can carry this oil in tiny droplets to the skin and into the nose, throat, and lungs.

A child can be poisoned by breathing fumes, such as **carbon monoxide**. Carbon monoxide is invisible—you can't see it or smell it. It is produced by equipment that burns fuel. Wood and gas fireplaces, gas water heaters, and gas ovens can make carbon monoxide if they are not working correctly or are not properly vented. A faulty furnace, a kerosene space heater, or a car motor running in an enclosed garage can produce carbon monoxide. Carbon monoxide poisoning causes rapid loss of responsiveness,

carbon monoxide
A deadly, invisible, odorless gas produced by equipment that burns fuel.

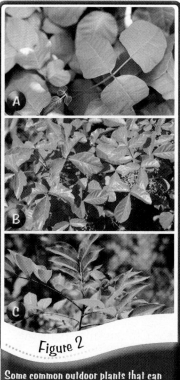

Figure 2

Some common outdoor plants that can cause a rash and sometimes an allergic reaction are (A) poison ivy, (B) poison oak, and (C) poison sumac.

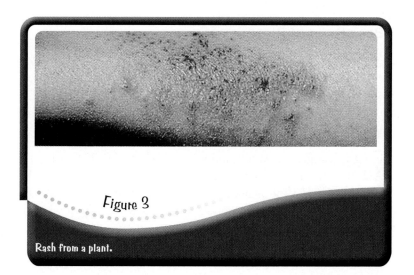

Figure 3

Rash from a plant.

sometimes preceded by a severe headache. It is often fatal. Carbon monoxide detectors are available. They can detect even a small amount of carbon monoxide in the air and warn you before the level becomes toxic.

A child can be poisoned by intentionally breathing in fumes from rubber cement or model glue.

What You Should Look For

Swallowed Poison

- Opened container of medicine or chemical
- Unusual odor from mouth or clothes
- Burns in and around the mouth indicating contact with a corrosive chemical
- Nausea or vomiting
- Abdominal pain or diarrhea
- Drowsiness
- Child is unresponsive

Contact with a Poisonous Plant

- Rash
- Itching
- Redness
- Blisters
- Swelling

Breathing of Poisonous Fumes

- A source of fumes that may or may not have an odor
- Change in behavior
- Change in appearance

What You Should Do

For any medical situation, follow the Six Steps of Pediatric First Aid. If your child has been poisoned, give first aid care. Call the Poison Help hotline as instructed in "What You Should Do." The medical professional who takes your call will tell you what to do next.

In the past, experts recommended that parents keep **syrup of ipecac** in the home as a poison treatment. In 2003, this recommendation was changed. Data showed that syrup of ipecac is not effective treatment for poisoning. Even if a child vomits after being given syrup of ipecac, too much poison can stay in the stomach. Do not use syrup of ipecac in a poisoning emergency.

syrup of ipecac A medicine that causes vomiting; it is not recommended for use in a poisoning emergency.

The Six Steps of Pediatric First Aid

1 Evaluate the Situation

Take a few seconds to look around. Evaluate the situation. Make sure the surroundings are safe. Find out who is involved and what happened.

2 Look and Listen for Signs of an Emergency

Look and listen for signs that your child's condition is serious or life threatening. Notice the ABCs (Appearance, Breathing, and Circulation). Always call emergency medical services (EMS) for life-threatening conditions. To call EMS, dial 911.

3 Check for Problems

Take a closer look and check your child for problems. Use the "What You Should Look For" sections to guide you. Figure out what is wrong, how serious it is, and what you should do next.

4 Act

Based on what is wrong, take action. Read the "What You Should Do" sections to be prepared. For a simple injury, you may only need to give first aid. For a serious condition, you may need to call EMS and give care until help arrives.

5 Follow Up

Be sure to follow up. Give any care or treatment that your child might need after the event.

6 Prevent

Take steps to prevent the illness or injury from happening again, if possible. Prevention is as important as first aid in caring for your child.

First Aid Care for Swallowed Poisons

 Gather information and remain calm. Try to determine the following:
- ► What the child swallowed
- ► How much was swallowed
- ► When it was swallowed
- ► The child's condition

 If the child is responsive, call the Poison Help hotline (1-800-222-1222). Have the child and the poison container with you. Follow the instructions from the Poison Help hotline professional.

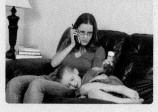

If the child is unresponsive, call EMS. Give CPR.

Place the child on his left side. Putting the child on his left side reduces the risk of choking in case the child vomits.

First Aid Care for Contact with a Poisonous Plant

 If a child's skin comes in contact with a poisonous plant, wash the area right away with soap. Flush with running water to rinse off the plant oil. If a child's eye or mouth is involved, flush with water.

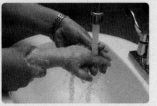

 Call the Poison Help hotline (1-800-222-1222) for what to do next.

First Aid Care for Breathing of Poisonous Fumes

 Remove the child from the area of the fumes and call EMS.

 If the child is responsive, call the Poison Help hotline (1-800-222-1222).

If the child is unresponsive, call EMS. Give CPR.

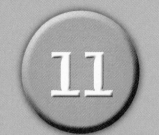

11

Burns

Burns

Introduction

burn An injury to the skin that results from heat, chemical, electrical, or radiation damage to the body.

A **burn** is an injury to the skin. Burns can be caused by heat, chemical, electrical, or radiation damage to the body (**Figure 1**). Sources of heat burns are hot water or steam, hot objects, and flames. Chemical burns are

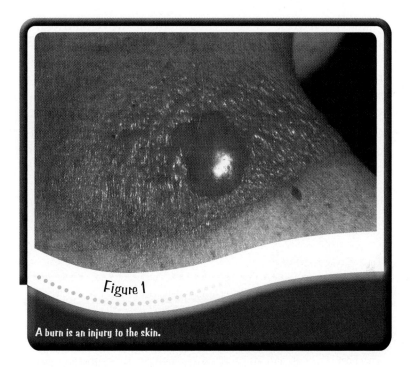

Figure 1

A burn is an injury to the skin.

caused by household chemicals or batteries. Electrical burns are caused by contact with electricity. Another type of burn is from radiation. The most common type of radiation burn is sunburn. Sunburn results from too much exposure to ultraviolet (UV) light. Burn injuries can be very painful. They may take a long time to heal. A serious burn injury can leave a child with long-term physical and emotional scars.

What You Should Know

Most burns to toddlers and preschoolers are scald injuries. Boiling water, hot foods, and steam can cause scald injuries. Keep your child out of the area where you are cooking. Always keep pot handles on top of the stove pointing toward the back. Be careful with hot cups of soup and coffee around children. Foods heated in the microwave can heat unevenly and cause burns. Never warm a baby's bottle in the microwave.

Burns can result from touching a hot object. Some hot objects found in the home are cooking surfaces, stoves, hot curling irons, and space heaters. An outdoor grill can stay hot enough to burn long after you are finished using it.

Flames often cause burns to children from 5 to 12 years old. Be sure you have smoke detectors in your home. Test them once a month to make sure they work. Teach your child to "drop and roll" in case his clothes catch on fire. Fires that create a lot of smoke can damage the airway and lungs. In case of a fire, teach your child to crawl under the smoke to get out of the building.

Chemicals, such as drain cleaner and household bleach, can cause burns. They destroy the skin that comes in direct contact with the chemical. The longer the chemical is in contact with the body, the more damage it does. Read labels on all household chemicals that you bring into your home. The label tells you if the product can cause burns. Store dangerous chemicals so that your child cannot

Did You Know?

sunscreen A chemical that bonds to the skin to prevent injury from UV light.

sunblock A barrier cream that prevents the UV light from reaching the skin.

People who have a history of one or more blistering sunburns during childhood or adolescence are two times more likely to develop skin cancer. Chronic exposure to UV light is the cause of most cases of skin cancer. More than half of a person's lifetime UV exposure is during childhood and adolescence. Protection from UV exposure reduces the risk for skin cancer. When children play outside, they should always wear sun-protective clothing and stay in the shade. Use sunscreen or sunblock. **Sunscreen** contains a chemical that bonds to the skin to prevent injury from UV light. **Sunblock** is a barrier cream that prevents the UV light from reaching the skin. Unlike burns from direct contact with hot surfaces, the irritation of the skin from sunburn takes time to develop.

Keep Your Child Safe

Bathwater or hot water from the faucet that is too hot can cause burns. Temperatures more than 120°F can cause serious injury to the skin within seconds. Set the thermostat on your hot water heater lower than 120°F. Consider installing antiscald devices on your bathtub faucet and shower head. Always test the temperature of your child's bathwater before putting the child in the tub.

get to them. When you use them, use and dispose of them carefully. The acid in batteries can cause a chemical burn. Keep new and used batteries away from children. Make sure your child can't take the batteries out of his toys. Be careful not to let him take batteries out of cell phones, portable phones, radios, and portable electronics.

Children are very curious. They can come upon electrical dangers, such as electrical outlets and wires, while exploring (**Figure 2**). Toddlers may try to place an object, such as a fork, into an electrical outlet. Babies may chew on wires. Usually children are knocked away by strong muscle contractions that occur after contact with electricity. However, these muscle contractions can make the child hold on to the object instead of being knocked away. This can cause more injury.

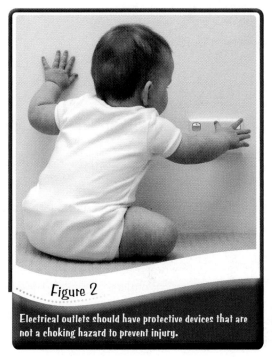

Figure 2

Electrical outlets should have protective devices that are not a choking hazard to prevent injury.

Injuries from electricity can range from a little reddening of the skin to severe damage to the body. The amount of damage depends on the amount of electricity. A child with an electrical burn may not have much damage on the surface of the skin but still have serious damage to the tissues underneath. Usually, electrical shock from a household current is not life threatening. Electrical shock, however, can cause the heart to stop. Be careful if the child who is injured by electricity is still in contact with the source of the electrical current. The electricity can flow to and hurt any person who touches the child.

The need for medical care depends upon the size, location, and depth of a burn. Larger and deeper burns are more serious injuries. Burns of the face, hands, feet, or genitals are more serious than burns in other locations of the body. Unfortunately, children often burn their faces, hands, feet, or genitals when they reach up to stovetops, touch hot appliances, or spill hot liquids in their laps. A burn that is a minor injury to an adult can be a serious injury for a young child.

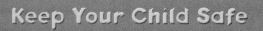

Keep Your Child Safe

Keep Your Child Safe from Burns

▸ Keep cribs and beds at a safe distance from radiators and electrical outlets.

▸ Cover outlets with child safety devices. (Be careful: Plastic plug covers can be a choking hazard if they fit too loosely or when you take them off to use the outlets.)

▸ Consider replacing standard electrical outlets with child-resistant electrical outlets.

▸ Don't let electrical cords hang over the edge of countertops or furniture.

▸ Check for damaged or frayed electrical cords.

▸ Don't use extension cords around babies and toddlers.

▸ Don't run electrical cords under rugs in areas of heavy traffic.

▸ Don't overload electrical circuits.

▸ Teach children that fire burns.

▸ Keep matches and lighters out of reach of children.

▸ Smoke detectors should be installed on each level of the house, in each bedroom, and outside each sleeping space.

▸ Test smoke detectors once a month.

▸ Have a fire escape plan. Designate a certain place for all children and adults to go. Hold practice fire drills regularly.

▸ Keep fire extinguishers where you can get to them. Have them checked every year to make sure they still work.

For more about how to protect your child from burns, go to http://www.cdc.gov/safechild/Burns/index.html.

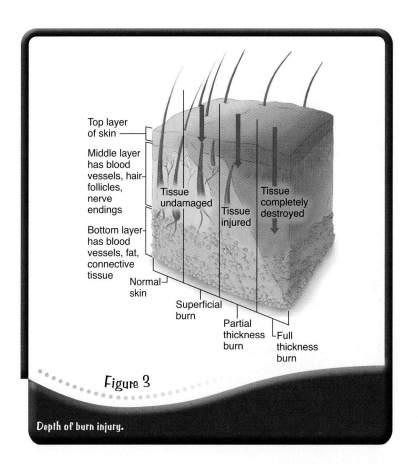

Top layer of skin

Middle layer has blood vessels, hair follicles, nerve endings

Bottom layer has blood vessels, fat, connective tissue

Tissue undamaged

Tissue injured

Tissue completely destroyed

Normal skin

Superficial burn

Partial thickness burn

Full thickness burn

Figure 3

Depth of burn injury.

To describe how big a burn is, compare the size of the burn with a familiar object (e.g., the burn is about the size of a quarter). Another way to describe the size of a burn is the percentage of the body part involved (e.g., about half of his back is burned). You can estimate the percent of the child's body involved in the burn by using the child's palm. The palm is about 1 percent of the total body surface. Add up the number of palm-sized areas of injured skin to estimate the percent of the body surface involved.

Medical providers describe the depth of a burn by using the following terms:

First-degree burns are minor burns on the top part of the skin. The skin is pink but does not blister. One example is a sunburn.

first-degree burns Burns that involve only the top part of the skin.

Second-degree burns are more serious and involve a deeper area. Symptoms are blisters, pain, and swelling. A second-degree burn needs medical care.

second-degree burns Burns that blister and involve a deeper thickness of the skin.

125

third-degree burns The most serious types of burns that involve deeper tissues under the skin.

Third-degree burns are the most serious types of burns. They involve deeper tissues under the skin. A third-degree burn can damage the full depth of skin, muscle, and nerves (**Figure 3**).

What You Should Look For

First-Degree Burn

- Pink or red skin
- Mild swelling, no blisters
- Mild to moderate pain

Second-Degree Burn

- Dark red or bright red skin
- Blisters
- Swelling
- Moderate to severe pain

Third-Degree Burn

- Red, raw, ash white, black, leathery, or charred skin
- Swelling
- Pain can be severe in the area around a third-degree burn, although there is little or no pain in the tissues that have a third-degree burn. This is because the nerves in that area have been destroyed.

Chemical Burn

- A change in the color of the skin
- Pain

Electrical Burn

- A source of electricity
- Red or white appearance to the skin that was in contact with the electricity

What You Should Do

For any medical situation, follow the Six Steps of Pediatric First Aid. If your child has a burn, give first aid care. Based on the type, location, depth, and severity of the burn, you will be able to decide if you need to call EMS or get medical care.

The Six Steps of Pediatric First Aid

 1 Evaluate the Situation

Take a few seconds to look around. Evaluate the situation. Make sure the surroundings are safe. Find out who is involved and what happened.

▼

 2 Look and Listen for Signs of an Emergency

Look and listen for signs that your child's condition is serious or life threatening. Notice the ABCs (Appearance, Breathing, and Circulation). Always call emergency medical services (EMS) for life-threatening conditions. To call EMS, dial 911.

▼

 3 Check for Problems

Take a closer look and check your child for problems. Use the "What You Should Look For" sections to guide you. Figure out what is wrong, how serious it is, and what you should do next.

▼

 4 Act

Based on what is wrong, take action. Read the "What You Should Do" sections to be prepared. For a simple injury, you may only need to give first aid. For a serious condition, you may need to call EMS and give care until help arrives.

▼

 **5 Follow Up**

Be sure to follow up. Give any care or treatment that your child might need after the event.

▼

6 Prevent

Take steps to prevent the illness or injury from happening again, if possible. Prevention is as important as first aid in caring for your child.

First Aid Care for Burns from Heat Sources, Including Sunburn

1 GET THE CHILD AWAY FROM THE SOURCE OF THE BURN.

▶ Remove the child from contact with the source of heat, sunshine, or whatever is causing the burn.

▶ If flames are present, smother them by using a blanket or rolling the child on the floor or ground. Keep the child from running because this fans the flames.

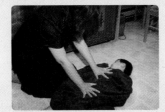

▶ Call EMS if the burn has injured areas that are raw, ash white, black, leathery, or charred (third-degree burns). Call EMS if the burn involves the child's face, hands, feet, or genitals. Call EMS if the burn is more than 10% of the body surface.

2 REMOVE BURNED CLOTHING.

▶ Any clothing or constricting jewelry should be removed before cooling.

▶ Take off burned clothing that isn't stuck to the skin. If clothing is stuck to the skin, cut around the stuck area and remove what you can. Leave the clothing that is stuck to the skin alone.

3 COOL THE BURN.

▶ Run cool water over the burned area. See the First Aid Tip for other ways to cool a burn. If the area is larger than the palm of the child's hand, you will need to limit the part that you cool at one time. Cool an area about three times the size of the child's palm so that the child doesn't get chilled. Cool one area for 1 to 2 minutes then move to another area.

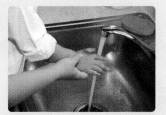

► Continue to cool the area until the pain stops or the child gets medical care.

4 **COVER THE BURN.**

► After the burn has cooled and the pain has stopped, cover it loosely with a dry bandage or clean cloth.

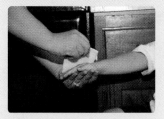

► Don't break any blisters. This could let germs get into the wound.

► **Never put grease (including butter or medical ointments) on the burn.** Grease holds in heat, which may make the burn worse. It also might interfere with medical treatment.

5 **KEEP THE CHILD FROM LOSING BODY HEAT.**

► Keep the child's body temperature normal. Cover unburned areas with a dry blanket if you think the child is getting chilled.

First Aid TIP

Ways to Cool a Burn

▷ Run a gentle flow of cool tap water over the burned area.

▷ Place the burned area in a container of cool water.

▷ Cover the burned area with a cold, wet towel if you can't put the area in cool water. Re-wet or replace the towel every 1 to 2 minutes.

First Aid Care
for Chemical Burns

 Stop the injury by removing the child from contact with the chemical.

 Brush off any dry chemical that is on the skin. Remove jewelry. Remove anything that might get too tight if the area swells.

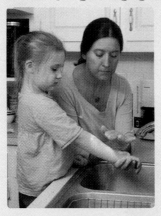

Call EMS.

Rinse the area of the body that was in contact with the chemical. Run a continuous gentle flow of fresh water over the entire affected area. Rinse for 15 to 20 minutes.

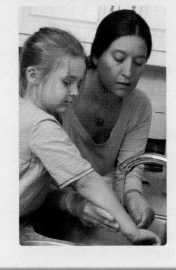

First Aid Care for Electrical Burns

 Be sure that the child is no longer connected to the source of the electricity. Turn off the power source before touching the child. If you are unable turn off the power source, push or pull the child away from the source of electricity with a thick dry cloth. For example, loop a dry towel around the child's feet. Another way is to push the child away with something made of wood. Examples are a broom handle or chair.

② Call EMS.

③ If the child is unresponsive, start CPR.

First Aid TIP

▶ Always cover ice before putting it on a burn. Putting ice directly on the skin can damage fragile tissues that remain.

▶ Don't apply burn ointments, petroleum jelly, margarine, toothpaste, or anything other than fresh cool water on a burn. A medical provider should prescribe any medicines that are used on a burn.

Keep blisters from breaking if you can. An unbroken blister helps prevent infection. When a blister breaks, germs can get into the damaged tissues and grow. After you finish cooling the burn, place a loose dressing over the blisters to try to protect them from breaking.

12

Heat- and Cold-Related Injuries

● Heat- and Cold-Related Injuries

Introduction

Children are more likely to be hurt by extremes of heat and cold than are adults. Children get chilled and overheated more quickly. They also are not as aware of dangers from heat and cold.

Problems from extremes of heat and cold are not just related to temperature. Wind, humidity, clothing, and length of exposure are involved. Wind chill may increase the risk of problems from cold. **Wind chill** is the difference between the actual temperature and how cold it feels because of the wind. Wind carries heat away from the body. This causes the body to cool more quickly than normal. Heat index may increase a child's risk of problems during hot weather. The **heat index** is the difference between the actual temperature and how hot it feels because of humidity and temperature. When the humidity is high, it is harder for sweat to evaporate. Without this evaporation, it is easier for the body to become overheated.

wind chill The difference between the actual temperature and how cold it feels because of the wind.

heat index The difference between the actual temperature and how hot it feels because of humidity and temperature.

Heat-Related Illness

What You Should Know

The body creates heat all the time. It makes more heat during exercise and sometimes during illness. The normal body temperature is 98.6° F. When the temperature is higher than that, the child has a fever. Temperatures higher than 106° F can cause permanent harm to the body.

When it is hot, the body makes sweat to cool itself. If the heat index is high, the sweat doesn't evaporate as fast. Cooling by sweating becomes less efficient. Some children do not sweat enough to cool themselves as well as other children. Wearing fabrics that trap sweat can limit cooling.

Usually, the first signs of too much body heat are nausea, headache, and confusion. If the body temperature does not go down, the child is at risk for brain damage and death. The most severe form of heat illness is **heatstroke**. Heatstroke is when the body's natural cooling system does not work normally. The body is not able to make sweat as usual. This causes a dangerous rise in body temperature.

heatstroke An illness that results when the body's natural cooling system does not work normally. The body is not able to make sweat as usual. This causes a dangerous rise in body temperature.

Heatstroke can develop quickly. A child with heatstroke will have a body temperature of 106° F or higher. When the sweat glands can no longer make moisture, the skin becomes dry and

flushing The skin on the child's face turns very red. Sometimes other areas of the body become red as well. Flushing can be a sign of a medical problem. Flushing is different from blushing. Blushing is usually a lighter pink or rose color. Blushing is associated with embarrassment.

heat exhaustion A condition that develops when children are exposed to hot temperatures for long periods of time. It often happens when they are actively playing and sweating. Heat exhaustion is caused by dehydration.

heat cramps Painful muscle spasms, usually in the legs and abdominal muscles. They are caused by dehydration.

dehydration A condition that results when the body doesn't have as much fluids as it needs. In hot weather this is caused by not drinking enough water to replace fluid that is lost through sweating.

hot. Often, the face and other parts of the body look **flushed** (red). The child breathes very fast. Then the child often becomes confused or unresponsive. Heatstroke is much more common in older people and athletes. However, children who are active in hot weather can have heatstroke. Heatstroke can occur in a baby who has too many clothes on and can't cool off enough.

Heat exhaustion can develop when children are exposed to hot temperatures for long periods of time. It often happens when they are actively playing and sweating. **Heat cramps** are painful muscle spasms. They are usually in the legs and abdominal muscles. Both heat exhaustion and heat cramps are caused by dehydration. **Dehydration** is when the body doesn't have as much fluid as it needs. In hot weather, this is caused by not drinking enough water to replace fluid that is lost through sweating (**Figure 1**).

A child who has heat exhaustion will be thirsty and sweating heavily. Pay attention to how often your child is urinating during hot conditions and what color the urine is. If the urine is dark and your child is not urinating at least once every 4 hours, he may be dehydrated. You can prevent dehydration by encouraging your child to drink more often, even if he only drinks a small amount at a time. A child who has heat exhaustion may feel weak, nauseated, and very tired. There is little or no elevation of the body temperature at this stage of heat illness. The child's tongue and mouth are likely to look dry. A child may have heat cramps with heat exhaustion.

What You Should Look For

When your child is in a hot environment, pay attention to the following:

- Heavy sweating for more than a short time or no sweating
- Looks and acts sick or more tired than expected; complains of nausea or headache

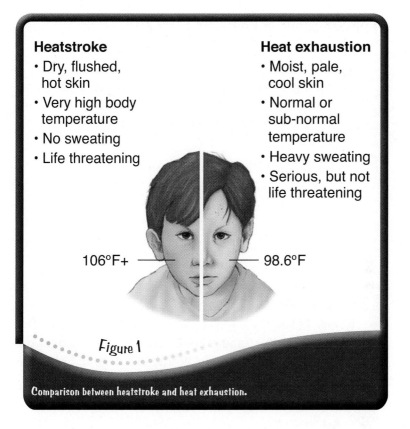

Heatstroke
- Dry, flushed, hot skin
- Very high body temperature
- No sweating
- Life threatening

Heat exhaustion
- Moist, pale, cool skin
- Normal or sub-normal temperature
- Heavy sweating
- Serious, but not life threatening

106°F+ ——— ——— 98.6°F

Figure 1

Comparison between heatstroke and heat exhaustion.

- Not urinating at least once every 4 hours and not drinking very often
- Skin is flushed, especially the face
- Confused
- Breathing faster than usual
- Body temperature is above normal

What You Should Do

For any medical situation, follow the Six Steps of Pediatric First Aid. If your child has a heat- or cold-related injury, give first aid care. Based on the instructions in "What You Should Do," you will know if you need to call EMS or get medical care.

The Six Steps of Pediatric First Aid

 **1** **Evaluate the Situation**

Take a few seconds to look around. Evaluate the situation. Make sure the surroundings are safe. Find out who is involved and what happened.

▼

 2 **Look and Listen for Signs of an Emergency**

Look and listen for signs that your child's condition is serious or life threatening. Notice the ABCs (Appearance, Breathing, and Circulation). Always call emergency medical services (EMS) for life-threatening conditions. To call EMS, dial 911.

▼

 3 **Check for Problems**

Take a closer look and check your child for problems. Use the "What You Should Look For" sections to guide you. Figure out what is wrong, how serious it is, and what you should do next.

▼

4 **Act**

Based on what is wrong, take action. Read the "What You Should Do" sections to be prepared. For a simple injury, you may only need to give first aid. For a serious condition, you may need to call EMS and give care until help arrives.

▼

 5 **Follow Up**

Be sure to follow up. Give any care or treatment that your child might need after the event.

▼

6 **Prevent**

Take steps to prevent the illness or injury from happening again, if possible. Prevention is as important as first aid in caring for your child.

Steps to Prevent Heatstroke and Heat Exhaustion

▶ Encourage your child to drink cool water frequently.

▶ Avoid strenuous activities during the midday hours when temperatures are usually the highest.

▶ Dress your child in lightweight, loose-fitting, sun-protective clothing in hot weather.

▶ Never leave a child alone in a car. Death from too much heat can occur in only a few minutes.

First Aid Care for Heatstroke

 Call EMS and cool the child right away. The best way to do this is to place wet, cool clothes, towels, or sheets on the body. If the child tolerates it, put ice packs or ice wrapped in a wet cloth in the armpits and groin. This will cool the blood that goes through the big blood vessels close to the skin in those areas.

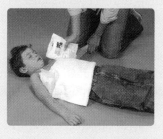

First Aid Care for Heat Exhaustion and Heat Cramps

1 Move the child to a cool place. If a cool place is not available, cool the child's body by using wet cool cloths. Continue to rinse and reapply cool cloths after they become warmed by contact with the body.

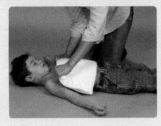

2 Encourage the child to drink lots of water. "Sports drinks" are not better than water.

Cold-Related Injuries

What You Should Know

hypothermia A dangerous condition that can develop when children are exposed to cold temperatures for long periods of time. The temperature deep within the body drops below 95°F.

frostbite Tissue damage caused by extreme cold.

frostnip The most common local cold injury. Although ice crystals form, the tissue doesn't actually freeze. The ice crystals melt once the body part is warmed. With frostnip there is not much tissue damage.

Hypothermia can develop when children are exposed to cold temperatures for long periods of time. This is a dangerous condition in which the temperature deep within the body drops below 95°F. Falling into cold water is a common cause. Another cause is being outside too long without proper clothing during cold weather. Body processes slow at these low temperatures. Tissue damage can occur. The outside temperature does not have to be below freezing for a child to have hypothermia.

Frostbite is tissue damage caused by extreme cold (**Figure 2**). A child's ears, face, hands, and feet are especially at risk. This is because the tissue in these areas is thin, exposed, or farther from the heart. **Frostnip** is the most common local cold injury. Although ice crystals form, the tissue doesn't actually freeze. The ice crystals melt once the body part is warmed. With frostnip there is not much tissue damage.

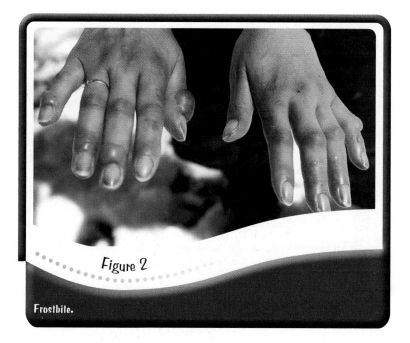

Figure 2

Frostbite.

What You Should Look For

- Body temperature is below normal
- Child is sluggish and may be unresponsive
- Injured skin with frostnip or frostbite looks cold and pale, and feels numb to the touch
- Injured skin may blister
- When body part is warmed, tissues that have been injured may have more blood in them than usual and may turn pink; if damage is severe, the body part may remain pale
- Mild to moderately damaged tissues hurt, tingle, and feel like they are burning

First Aid Care for Hypothermia

 Bring the child into a warm place and call EMS. Until you can get to a warm room, bring the child close to someone else's warm body.

2 Take off the cold wet clothes and replace them with warm dry ones.

3 Wrap the child in a blanket.

First Aid Care for Frostbite and Frostnip

 Take the child to a warm room and call EMS. Until you can get to a warm room, place cold body parts close to warm body areas. For example, tuck cold hands into the armpits.

 Remove any wet clothes, including shoes and socks. Cover the areas with clean, warm, and dry coverings.

 Don't break any blisters that may be present. Cover those that have broken with gauze.

4 Let the cold-injured part return to normal body temperature slowly.

5 If toes or fingers are cold damaged, put dry gauze between the toes or fingers to keep them from rubbing each other.

6 Call your medical provider. Your child may need medical care.

Keep Your Child Safe

Steps to Prevent Hypothermia, Frostbite, and Frostnip

When your child is in a cold environment, do the following:

▶ Dress your child to prevent problems from the cold. Your child may need to wear mittens, a hat, and a warm coat. In very cold climates, your child may need insulated and water-repellent boots and snow pants.

▶ Bring your child indoors right away if she complains of a cold, numb, tingling, or painful area on her body.

Eye Injuries

Introduction

An **eye injury** includes injury to the eye, eyelid, and area around the eye. Common eye injuries are caused by scratches, cuts, and foreign bodies. Other common

> **eye injury** Injury to the eye, eyelid, and area around the eye.

eye injuries come from burns, chemicals, and blows to the eye. The main concern when a child has an eye injury is possible damage to the child's vision. Eye injuries are the most common and preventable causes of blindness.

According to the National Society to Prevent Blindness, about 33% of vision loss in children younger than 10 years old is caused by trauma to the eye. Some activities that often cause

eye trauma Any injury to the eye. **eye trauma** are baseball, basketball, hockey, and sports that involve rackets. Other activities are bicycling, boxing, archery, darts, and BB guns. Fingernails, toys, and chemicals are also common causes of eye injury. Each year, toys and home playground equipment cause more than 11,000 injuries to young eyes.

What You Should Know

Take steps to prevent eye injuries before they happen. Look around your home for sharp or pointed objects. Remove or put them away where young children cannot play with them. Remember that a common household object, such as pencil, knife, or fork, can injure a child if he falls on it. Don't let older children run and play while carrying a sharp or pointed object.

Toys are designed to be used by children within a certain age range. Don't let young children play with toys designed for older children. Examine your child's toys for sharp edges or pointed parts. Avoid toys that fly or shoot. Keep BB guns away from children. Check your child's play areas and equipment to make sure they are safe. Don't allow playing with sticks. Make sure your child wears the proper eye-protective equipment when playing sports.

Keep dangerous household chemicals, such as cleaners, paints, and glues, in a locked cabinet. Read labels for all chemicals that you buy to understand which products will cause burns or problems if splashed into the eye. Keep your child out of the work area when handling these products.

What You Should Look For

- Double vision
- Decrease in vision
- Sensitivity to light
- Redness or swelling

- Pain when moving the eye in any direction
- Blood in the eye
- Dizziness
- Numbness
- Inability to open eye after trauma

If your child has any of these problems, get medical care right away.

What You Should Do

For any medical situation, follow the Six Steps of Pediatric First Aid. If your child has an eye injury, give first aid care. Based on the type of injury, you will be able to decide if you need to call EMS or get medical care.

The Six Steps of Pediatric First Aid

1 Evaluate the Situation

Take a few seconds to look around. Evaluate the situation. Make sure the surroundings are safe. Find out who is involved and what happened.

▼

2 Look and Listen for Signs of an Emergency

Look and listen for signs that your child's condition is serious or life threatening. Notice the ABCs (Appearance, Breathing, and Circulation). Always call emergency medical services (EMS) for life-threatening conditions. To call EMS, dial 911.

▼

3 Check for Problems

Take a closer look and check your child for problems. Use the "What You Should Look For" sections to guide you. Figure out what is wrong, how serious it is, and what you should do next.

▼

4 Act

Based on what is wrong, take action. Read the "What You Should Do" sections to be prepared. For a simple injury, you may only need to give first aid. For a serious condition, you may need to call EMS and give care until help arrives.

▼

 5 Follow Up

Be sure to follow up. Give any care or treatment that your child might need after the event.

▼

 6 Prevent

Take steps to prevent the illness or injury from happening again, if possible. Prevention is as important as first aid in caring for your child.

First Aid Care for Chemical Injury to the Eye

 ❶ Wear protective gloves if available. Flush the chemical from the eye with lukewarm water right away.

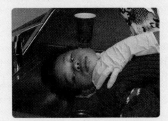

❷ Position your child's head over the sink with the injured eye down. This will prevent the rinse water from contaminating the other eye.

❸ Hold the injured eye open with your fingers and flush with water for 15 minutes.

❹ Rinse from the inside (nose side) of the eye toward the outside (ear side) of the eye. You may need to securely hold the child still.

 ❺ Have someone call the Poison Help hotline (1-800-222-1222) while you flush the eye.

Chemicals get into children's eyes most often from products in spray bottles, such as household cleaners and pesticides. A chemical burn to the eye requires immediate first aid treatment to prevent damage to the cornea. The **cornea** is the transparent outer covering of the eyeball. Eye damage can occur quickly—in less than 5 minutes. Certain chemicals can cause rapid and severe damage. The eye may not appear red, but vision may be threatened.

cornea The transparent outer covering of the eyeball.

First Aid Care for Penetrating Injury to the Eye

 Call EMS.

 Penetrating eye injuries often include cuts or open wounds in the eye. Try to cover the injured eye with an eye shield, paper cup, or even cardboard folded into a cone. If your child strongly resists covering the eye, do not insist.

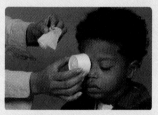

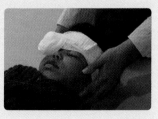 Keep your child as quiet as possible. The best position is for the child to lie still and be flat on his back. Don't force the child to lie in this position if he resists. Never try to remove a foreign object that is penetrating the eye. This may cause more damage. Never apply pressure to the eye. Don't apply any medicine.

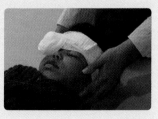

First Aid Care for Foreign Object in the Eye

 A foreign body can be any material that gets into the eye. Examples of a foreign body are dust, sand, or an insect. Wear medical gloves if available. Pull down the child's lower eyelid to look at the inner surface while the child looks up. A speck of dirt can usually be removed with a clean wet gauze or handkerchief.

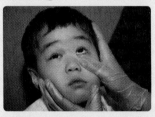

 Gently grasp the upper lid and pull it out and down over the lower eyelid. This causes the eye to make tears. Tears may help dislodge the object.

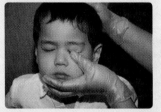

 If the object is still there, flush the eye with water. Position your child's head over a sink, injured eye down. Hold the eye open with your fingers. Use an unbreakable cup to rinse from the inside (nose side) of the eye toward the outside (ear side) of the eye. Don't apply medicine.

Your child should get medical care if the eye continues to tear or be red or painful. The foreign body might have scratched the cornea. A scratched cornea can only be confirmed by a professional with a special dye and medical equipment.

146

Did You Know

Foreign objects that often get in the eye are eyelashes, dirt, insects, and bits of sand. These can cause discomfort, redness, and tearing of the eyes. If your child has a foreign object in her eye, rubbing the eye can scratch the cornea. This is a very painful injury. It can lead to a serious infection. Covering an injured eye may reduce some of the pain, but it will not heal the injury. Don't force your child to cover her eye if she resists. That could cause more damage to the eye if there is something under the eyelid or stuck in the eye.

First Aid Care for Cut on the Eye or Lid

1 Keep the child sitting down.

2 Wear medical gloves if available.

3 If the child will tolerate it, cover the injured eye with a gauze pad and bandage loosely. Don't try to flush the eye with water or apply pressure to the injured eyelid. Don't put any medicine in the eye.

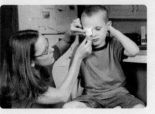

4 Get medical care.

147

First Aid Care for Blow to the Eye

 Gently place an ice pack or a cold pack wrapped in a wet cloth on the injured eye for 10 to 15 minutes to control swelling and reduce pain.

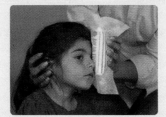

 A black eye, redness, pain, or blurred vision might mean that the eye is damaged. It may mean that the eye is swelling inside. Don't apply medicine.

 Get medical care as soon as possible.

148

14

Oral Injuries

● Teeth

Introduction

Most children start getting teeth at about 6 months old. A child who is 3 years old will have a full set of primary teeth. **Primary teeth** are also called

primary teeth Also known as baby teeth, primary teeth usually begin to grow at about 6 months old. Most children have a full set of primary teeth at about age 3.

"baby" teeth. Primary teeth serve a number of purposes. They are involved in speech development. They help the child to chew properly and get good nutrition. They also act as space savers for permanent teeth. When a child is about 6 years old, her jaw will begin to grow to make room for **permanent**, or "adult," teeth. From the ages of 6 to 12 years, children will lose primary teeth. Permanent teeth will replace them.

permanent teeth Teeth that develop at about 6 years old to replace primary teeth. By age 21 years, usually all 32 of the permanent teeth have erupted.

What You Should Know

A permanent tooth that is knocked out is a dental emergency that needs first aid care right away. A child with a knocked-out tooth needs to be seen by a dentist as soon as possible. A permanent tooth that is knocked out should be placed back into the socket. This gives the tooth a greater chance of survival. Primary, or baby, teeth should not be reinserted.

What You Should Look For

- A missing tooth in the child's mouth
- Bleeding from the mouth
- Child is very upset

What You Should Do

The Six Steps of Pediatric First Aid

 **1** Evaluate the Situation

Take a few seconds to look around. Evaluate the situation. Make sure the surroundings are safe. Find out who is involved and what happened.

▼

2 Look and Listen for Signs of an Emergency

Look and listen for signs that your child's condition is serious or life threatening. Notice the ABCs (Appearance, Breathing, and Circulation). Always call emergency medical services (EMS) for life-threatening conditions. To call EMS, dial 911.

▼

3 Check for Problems

Take a closer look and check your child for problems. Use the "What You Should Look For" sections to guide you. Figure out what is wrong, how serious it is, and what you should do next.

▼

4 Act

Based on what is wrong, take action. Read the "What You Should Do" sections to be prepared. For a simple injury, you may only need to give first aid. For a serious condition, you may need to call EMS and give care until help arrives.

▼

5 Follow Up

Be sure to follow up. Give any care or treatment that your child might need after the event.

▼

6 Prevent

Take steps to prevent the illness or injury from happening again, if possible. Prevention is as important as first aid in caring for your child.

First Aid Care for Knocked-Out Permanent Tooth

1 Position the child so that bleeding doesn't cause him to choke.

2 Wear medical gloves if available. Control any bleeding.

3 Try to find the tooth. If you find the tooth, don't handle it by the roots.

4 If the tooth is dirty, rinse it gently with water. Don't scrub or use antiseptic on the tooth.

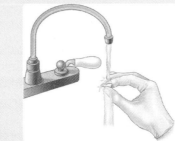

5 Gently place the tooth back in the socket. If the child is able to assist, ask him to hold the tooth in place with a finger or tissue. Don't try to reinsert a primary (baby) tooth.

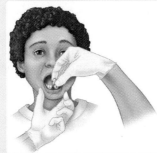

6 If you cannot reinsert the tooth, place the tooth in a glass of milk. If milk is not available, wrap the tooth in a cold wet cloth.

7 Get medical care right away. For best results, the child should be seen by a dentist within 1 hour of the time the tooth was knocked out.

First Aid TIP

If you can't find a knocked-out tooth, it is still important to have your child seen by a dentist as soon as possible. The tooth may be knocked up into the gums. This can happen with either a primary or permanent tooth.

Toothaches

What You Should Know

Toothaches may be dental emergencies. However, sometimes toothaches are caused by reasons that are not dental emergencies. Some of these reasons are eruption of teeth, sores in the mouth, earaches, and sinus infections. Your child should be seen by a dentist or medical provider to identify the source of the pain.

What You Should Look For

- Complaints of pain
- Drooling
- If the child is old enough, ask him to point to what hurts; ask him to show you which tooth hurts

First Aid Care for Toothaches

 Have the child rinse his mouth with warm water.

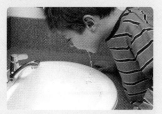

 Use dental floss to remove any food that might be caught between the teeth.

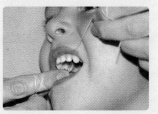

 Look for swelling or a "pimple" around the tooth. This may be a sign of a dental abscess.

4 See if the tooth is loose.

5 Your child may need to see a dentist or medical provider.

First Aid TIP

If your child complains of a toothache, a medical provider may be able to identify what is causing the problem. Sometimes an infection or mouth sores may feel like a toothache to a child. If these are not the problem, your child needs to be seen by a dentist. If your child has any swelling in the mouth or on the face, get medical care as soon as possible.

Bites

What You Should Know

A child may bite her lip or tongue while eating or during a fall. Even small cuts on the lip or tongue can cause a large amount of bleeding. This may make it hard to figure out the size of the injury.

What You Should Look For

- A hole in the lip or tongue that is the size and shape of a tooth mark
- Bleeding

First Aid Care for Bites to the Tongue or Lips

 Wear medical gloves if available.

 Have the child rinse with water so that you can identify where the injury is.

 Apply pressure with a piece of gauze or cloth to stop the bleeding.

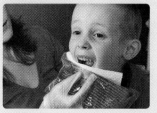

4 Apply ice or a cold pack wrapped in cloth or towel if there is any swelling.

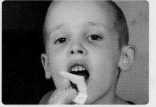

5 Injuries that go all the way through the lip or that cut across the edge of the tongue should be seen by a medical provider. These injuries may need stitches.

What Can I Do to Keep My Child Safe?

● What Can I Do to Keep My Child Safe?

Introduction

Parents and caregivers want to keep their children safe. But many times there may be dangers in the home or play area that they don't recognize. Take a few minutes to read the important tips in this chapter. Chances are you will find a few new ways to help make your child's environment safer.

As a parent or caregiver, you have the important task of nurturing and caring for your child. Children cannot always make good decisions about their own health and safety. This puts them at greater risks for injuries, such as burns, falls, choking, and poisoning (**Figure 1**). One of the most important roles of a parent or caregiver is to protect your child from harm. Prevention is as important as first aid in caring for your child.

What You Should Know

Being aware of dangers in your child's environment is the key to keeping your child safe. Children are more prone to certain injuries based on their age and development. Babies explore objects by putting them in their mouth. Toddlers are impulsive and try to touch everything within reach. Preschoolers try to imitate adult behavior. School-age children have more independence when playing outside and at school. Parents and caregivers must pay attention to safety risks at each stage of their child's development (**Table 1**).

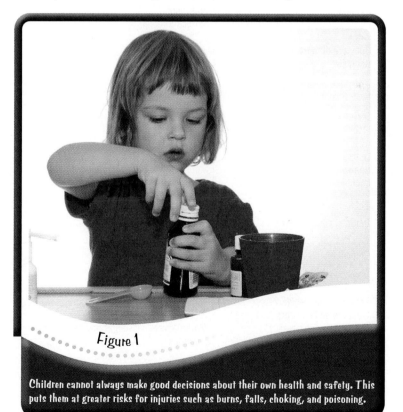

Figure 1

Children cannot always make good decisions about their own health and safety. This puts them at greater risks for injuries such as burns, falls, choking, and poisoning.

Table 1 Common Injuries Related to a Child's Developmental Level

Developmental Characteristics	Common Injuries
Infant—Age 0 to 1 Year	
Increasing mobility Uses mouth to explore objects Reaches for and pulls objects Unaware of dangers Cannot understand "no"	Burns Choking Drowning Falls Suffocation
Toddler—Age 1 to 2½ Years	
Travels in cars Masters walking, running, climbing Explores almost everything with mouth Begins to imitate behaviors Investigates everything within reach Curious about never-before-seen item Unaware of most dangers Impulsive	Burns Choking Drowning Falls Motor vehicle passenger and pedestrian injuries Poisoning Suffocation
Preschooler—Age 2½ to 5 Years	
Travels in cars Mobility leads to increased independence Learns to ride tricycle Unaware of many dangers Might favor real tools, gadgets, appliances rather than toys Fascinated with fire Imitates adult behavior	Burns Choking Drowning Falls Motor vehicle passenger and pedestrian injuries Poisoning
School-Aged—Age 5 Years and Up	
Travels in cars Walks alone Seeks independence Wants to be like peers Likes to be with peers Needs increased physical activity Dangers do not always seem real Increased independence can mean less supervision Plays sports	Bicycle injuries Burns Falls Firearm injuries Motor vehicle passenger and pedestrian injuries

What You Should Look For

The first step to creating a safe environment for your child is to identify possible dangers. Inspect every room in your home. Inspect everywhere your child may visit or play. Keep in mind specific risks based on your child's age and development. Are there refrigerator magnets that your toddler could choke on? Could your preschooler crawl up on the counter and reach medicines in a high cabinet? Does your toddler have access to an older child's games with small pieces?

Also check the garage and outdoor areas. Are power tools plugged in and waiting for your school-age child to use? Could your child get in the car and take it out of gear? Is the outdoor play equipment safe from sharp edges? Does your child wear her bike helmet every time she gets on her bike?

What You Should Do

Taking steps to keep your child safe will reduce the likelihood that you will need to use your first aid skills. However, if your child has a first aid emergency, it is important to follow the Six Steps of Pediatric First Aid.

The Six Steps of Pediatric First Aid

1 Evaluate the Situation

Take a few seconds to look around. Evaluate the situation. Make sure the surroundings are safe. Find out who is involved and what happened.

▼

2 Look and Listen for Signs of an Emergency

Look and listen for signs that your child's condition is serious or life threatening. Notice the ABCs (Appearance, Breathing, and Circulation). Always call emergency medical services (EMS) for life-threatening conditions. To call EMS, dial 911.

▼

3 Check for Problems

Take a closer look and check your child for problems. Use the "What You Should Look For" sections to guide you.

Figure out what is wrong, how serious it is, and what you should do next.

4 **Act**

Based on what is wrong, take action. Read the "What You Should Do" sections to be prepared. For a simple injury, you may only need to give first aid. For a serious condition, you may need to call EMS and give care until help arrives.

5 **Follow Up**

Be sure to follow up. Give any care or treatment that your child might need after the event.

▼

6 **Prevent**

Take steps to prevent the illness or injury from happening again, if possible. Prevention is as important as first aid in caring for your child.

What You Should Do

Tips to Keep Your Child Safe in the Kitchen

- Install childproof latches on all cabinet drawers and doors.
- Don't store cleaning supplies, bug sprays, and dishwasher detergent under the sink. Keep them in a place your child can't reach.
- Store all vitamins and medicines in a locked cabinet. This includes prescription drugs as well as over-the-counter medicine, such as acetaminophen and aspirin.
- Place the garbage can behind a cabinet door with a childproof latch.
- Remember that alcohol can be poisonous to a child. Keep beer, wine, and all alcohol stored out of reach.
- Look at the refrigerator magnets. If a child can get something entirely in his mouth, it's a choking hazard.
- Keep chairs and step stools away from the stove.
- Keep your child away from the cooking area when you are using the stove or sharp knives.

- Turn pot handles toward the back of the stove when you are cooking. Try to cook on the back burners when possible.
- Store glass objects out of your child's reach.
- Keep plastic garbage bags, plastic wrap, and sandwich bags away from your child.
- Unplug small appliances and store them in a safe place.
- Look for electrical cords or telephone wires that could be dangerous.
- Put matches and lighters in a locked cabinet.
- Be careful with hot cups of soup and coffee.
- Don't heat a baby's bottle in the microwave. It could have hot spots and cause burns.
- Supervise your child when eating. Children should not run and play with food in their mouths.
- Store food that is a choking hazard, such as nuts or grapes, away from small children. See *Chapter 3: Breathing Problems* for a detailed list of food to avoid in children younger than 4 years.

What You Should Do

Tips to Keep Your Child Safe in the Bedroom

- Never leave your baby alone for even a second on a changing table. Have everything ready before you start to change a diaper.
- Never leave your baby alone for even a second on a bed. Even if he is asleep, he could wake up and roll off.
- Keep side rails up on the crib.
- Select safe nursery furniture. Be especially careful if you are buying used items. All painted cribs, bassinets, and high chairs should be free of lead paint risks (made after 1978). Periodically check crib, playpen, and high chair recalls, even if you bought them new. More than 2 million cribs were recalled in 2008.
- Reduce the risk of sudden infant death syndrome (SIDS) by keeping soft pillows, stuffed animals, and soft bedding out of the crib. Don't use crib bumper pads. See "Tips to Reduce the Risk of SIDS."

- Look for strings or ribbons that might be dangerous. Clip them off hanging mobiles and crib toys. Remove drawstrings from your child's clothes. Don't put a pacifier on a string around a baby's neck. Don't put a necklace or ribbon around a baby's neck.

- Check blinds and curtains to make sure cords are tied up. Whenever possible, use cordless window coverings.

- Secure chest of drawers to the wall so if a child crawls in a drawer, it won't fall over on him.

- Make sure toy chests or other storage containers have a lid support to keep the lid from slamming down on the child's hands. Toy chests should not lock.

- Install operable window guards if the bedroom is on the second floor. Install window guards for any window where your child might push out the screen and crawl out. Do not put furniture, including the crib, near a window.

- Check to make sure all toys are age appropriate for your child.

- Choose pajamas that are made of flame-retardant material.

- Place all electrical cords so your child can't get to them. This includes cords on clocks, radios, and lamps.

- Keep nightlights from touching curtains, bedspreads, or other fabric.

- Take a look at other bedrooms where your child might go. Secure medicines, coins, scissors, and any small or sharp objects.

What You Should Do

Tips to Keep Your Child Safe in the Bathroom

- Install child-resistant latches on all cabinet drawers and doors.

- Don't store cleaning supplies under the sink. Keep them in a place your child can't reach.

- Store all medicine bottles in a locked cabinet. This includes prescription drugs as well as over-the-counter medicine, such as acetaminophen, aspirin, and vitamins.

- Check for poison hazards in the bathroom. Store them out of reach or in a locked cabinet. Some poisons found in bathrooms are mouthwash, perfume, hair dye, hairspray, nail polish, and nail polish remover.

- Store sharp tools, such as razor blades and nail scissors, so that your child cannot get to them.
- Avoid plastic-backed adhesive bandages. They are a choking hazard. Use fabric adhesive bandages instead.
- Never leave a child unsupervised in a bathroom. A child can drown in a toilet.
- Unplug the hair dryer, curling iron, and electric razor when they are not being used.
- Make sure outlets in the bathroom have grounded circuit breakers.
- Supervise your child in the tub at all times. If you have to answer the phone or the doorbell, take your child with you.
- Reduce the risk of burns by setting the thermostat on the water heater below 120° F.
- Monitor your child if you are interrupted when using cleaning supplies in the bathroom, such a toilet cleaner or bleach.

What You Should Do

Tips to Keep Your Child Safe in the Laundry Room and Garage

Poison Hazards

Keep the following stored in a locked cabinet or where your child cannot get to them:

- Cleaning products
- Laundry detergent
- Stain removers and bleach
- Rust remover
- Lawn care supplies, such as weed killer
- Bug spray, rat poison
- Fertilizer
- Paints and paint thinner
- Petroleum products, such as gasoline, kerosene, lighter fluid
- Antifreeze, windshield washer fluid
- Batteries, both new and used

Dangerous Tools

Make sure your child cannot access sharp or dangerous tools, such as:

- Drills
- Power saws
- Lawnmower
- Weed eater, hedge clippers
- Chain saw
- Screw drivers
- Axe, hatchet, hand saws
- Nail and staple guns
- Fishing gear, such as hooks and lures

Other Hazards

- Take your car keys out of the car and keep them where your child can't get them.
- Keep your car locked. Your child could get in the car and take it out of gear.
- Install only garage door openers with sensors. A mechanical garage door may crush a child.

What You Should Do

Tips to Keep Your Child Safe Throughout the House

- Install safety gates and operable guards where needed to protect your child from falls.
- Install door knob covers on exterior doors so that a young child won't be able to leave the house.
- Make sure the television is secured so that your child cannot pull it over on himself. Don't let young children operate electronic equipment.
- Caution anyone who smokes cigarettes or other tobacco products about the dangers to your child. Tobacco products can be toxic if a child eats them. Secondhand smoke may cause health problems in a child. Keep matches and lighters away from children.
- Buy a fire extinguisher for your home. Keep one in the kitchen and in any room with a furnace or fireplace. Have fire extinguishers checked once a year to make sure they still work.

- Install smoke alarms in your home, particularly in sleeping areas. Check the batteries once a month.

- Have a fire escape plan for your family. Designate a certain place for all children and adults to go. Hold practice fire drills regularly.

- Consider installing a carbon monoxide detector.

- Remove all guns from your home, if possible. Handguns are especially dangerous. If you choose to keep a gun at home, store it unloaded in a locked place. Lock and store the ammunition in a separate place. Find out if there are guns at other places your child might go to visit or play. Speak up and make sure all guns are properly stored before allowing your child to be there.

- Check for dangers in the homes of friends or relatives where your child may play. Homes with no children or older children may have many hazards. Common hazards are poisons, places where your child might fall, pools, and guns.

- Keep visitors' purses and coats away from small children. They could contain poisoning or choking hazards, such as medicine, small candies, or small objects.

- Review the list of poisons frequently found in the home in *Chapter 10: Poisoning.*

- Keep the Poison Help hotline number by every phone and store it in your cellular phone (1-800-222-1222).

What You Should Do

Tips to Keep Your Child Safe During Winter

- Have your heating system and fireplaces inspected once a year. This will help prevent carbon monoxide poisoning and fires.

- Don't use a portable grill for a heat source indoors. Never run a gasoline generator inside. They produce deadly levels of carbon monoxide quickly.

- Teach your child that fires are dangerous. Don't let her play with candles, matches, or lighters.

- Use a fire screen around the fireplace. Supervise children around open flames at all times.

- Put barriers around space heaters, wood stoves, and kerosene heaters to protect your child from burns. Keep these heaters away from furniture or curtains.

- Dress your child to prevent problems from the cold. Your child may need to wear mittens, a hat, and a warm coat. In very cold climates, she may need insulated and water-repellent boots and snow pants. Dressing your child in layers of clothing will help her stay warm while giving her the flexibility to take off a layer if she gets too hot.
- Bring your child indoors right away if she complains of a cold, numb, tingling, or painful area on her body.

What You Should Do

Tips to Keep Your Child Safe During Summer

- Encourage your child to drink cool water frequently.
- Avoid strenuous activities during the midday hours when temperatures are usually the highest.
- Dress your child in lightweight, loose-fitting, sun-protective clothing in hot weather.
- Never leave a child alone in a car. Death from too much heat can occur in only a few minutes.
- Children are outside more during the summer. See "Keep Your Child Safe Outside" and "Keep Your Child Safe Around Water" for more tips.

What You Should Do

Tips to Keep Your Child Safe Around Water

- Never leave a child alone near a pool or body of water. Even a small lily pond can be a drowning risk for a toddler.
- Practice touch supervision with young children. This means that the child is never more than an arm's reach from an adult.
- Fence in your pool or hot tub on all sides, separated from the house and the rest of the yard. Make sure that any pool or hot tub near where your child plays is fenced. Check fence gates to make sure they are locked.
- Children should learn to swim when they are developmentally ready.
- Put a life jacket on your child when he rides in a boat, is on a pier, or is around a body of water.

- Make sure children are always supervised when swimming, even if they swim well. Swimming ability cannot "drown-proof" a child of any age.
- Empty bathtubs, buckets, and other containers immediately after use.

What You Should Do

Tips to Keep Your Child Safe in and Around Cars

- Use a car safety seat for every trip—even short ones. Always place the car safety seat in the rear seat of your car.

- Select a car safety seat that fits your child's size and age. Read the instruction manual that comes with the seat. Also look at the section on child seats in the owner's manual for your car. Not every car safety seat is a good fit in every car.

- Keep up-to-date on recalls for your car safety seat. Go online to http://www-odi.nhtsa.dot.gov/recalls/childseat.cfm to see if a safety seat has been recalled.

- Make sure the car safety seat is installed correctly. It shouldn't move more than 1 inch side to side or back to front. If it does, it's either not installed correctly or needs to be tightened. Child safety seat inspection stations will inspect your seat for free. A technician will show you how to install your seat and use it. To find a location near you, go to http://www.seatcheck.org or call toll-free at 1-866-SEATCHECK (1-866-732-8243).

- Make sure the straps are snug enough when putting your child in the car safety seat. Try the pinch test: the strap should be too tight to pinch between your fingers.

- Infants should ride facing the rear of the car until they reach the weight or height limit set by the manufacturer. These limits can be found in the instruction manual or on a label on the side of the seat. Never place a rear-facing seat in front of an air bag.

- Use a booster seat on every trip for a child who has outgrown her car safety seat. This is usually when the child is at least 4 years old and about 40 or more pounds. A child should use a booster seat until the seat belt fits correctly, usually when she is at least 4 feet 9 inches tall and usually between the ages of 8 and 12 years.

- Be a good role model. Wear your seat belt at all times.
- A car safety seat will need to be replaced if it was installed in the car at the time of a moderate to severe crash. Insurance will sometimes cover a replacement.
- Lock the car doors before driving. Keep the car doors locked when the car is not in use. Always remove the keys when you get out of the car.
- Never leave a child alone in the car. Cases have been reported where an adult was distracted and forgot that a baby was asleep in the back seat. Children can overheat and die quickly. Put your purse, cell phone, or briefcase in the back seat with the baby. Then you won't forget and leave the car without her.
- Make sure children keep their arms, legs, and heads inside a moving vehicle. Be cautious of electric windows.
- Don't allow your child to ride in the back of a pick-up truck.
- Keep young children from playing in driveways or near busy streets.
- Always walk behind the car before backing down a driveway. You may not see a child in the rearview mirror.
- Teach your child to follow safety rules when crossing the street.

Get more information about selecting, installing, and using car safety seats online at http://www.healthychildren.org/carseatguide.

What You Should Do

Tips to Keep Your Child Safe on a Bicycle

- Don't carry a child younger than 12 months on a bicycle. This includes carrying a child in a backpack or front pack.
- Use an approved child bike carrier.
- Children from 1 to 4 years old wearing a helmet may ride in a rear-mounted seat.
- Avoid riding in busy streets with your child.
- All children should wear bicycle helmets. Select an approved helmet and make sure it is the right size.
- Be a good role model and always wear your helmet.
- Supervise where your child rides his bicycle. Younger children should ride in protected areas. Examples are on bike paths or in parks.

- Don't let your child ride his bike after dark.
- Don't allow your child to ride a passenger on his bike.

What You Should Do

Tips to Keep Your Child Safe Outside

- Know what type of plants, trees, and berries grow in your child's play area. Keep your child away from poisonous ones.
- Check the surface under play equipment. There should be cushioning material that will absorb the force of a fall, such as a safety rubber mat. Other acceptable materials are 12 inches of sand, sawdust, or wood chips.
- Home trampolines are very dangerous. They are the cause of thousands of injuries every year in children. Children over the age of 6 should only be allowed on a trampoline as part of a supervised athletic program, such as gymnastics.
- Teach your child to stay away from wild animals and unfamiliar pets. See "Keep Your Children Safe from Dog Bites by Teaching Them How to Behave Around Dogs" in *Chapter 9: Bites and Stings.*
- Help protect your child from insect stings. See "How to Protect Your Child from Insect Stings" in *Chapter 9: Bites and Stings.*
- Keep your child indoors when someone is operating a lawn mower outside. A child should never be a passenger on a riding lawnmower. A child should be at least 12 years old to mow the grass with a push lawnmower; a child should be at least 16 years old to operate a riding lawn mower.
- Children under 16 years of age who are not licensed to drive a car should not operate ATVs, and no child should be a passenger on an ATV. ATVs should never be operated on paved roads.
- Remove doors from refrigerators or freezers that have been discarded outside.
- Don't let children light or play with fireworks, including sparklers. Sparklers burn at very high temperatures. Many fireworks injuries to children are caused by sparklers.
- Don't leave ladders propped up against the house. Ladders invite children to climb.

What You Should Do

Tips to Reduce the Risk of SIDS

Sudden infant death syndrome (SIDS) is an unexplained death in babies younger than 1 year old. It is not known exactly what causes SIDS. Experts agree that doing the following reduces the risk of SIDS:

- Put your baby on her back to sleep. Putting the baby to sleep on her side is not recommended.

- Use a firm mattress.

- Don't place soft toys or objects in the baby's bed. Don't place loose blankets around or on the baby during sleep. Consider using a sleeper as an alternative to blankets. If using a thin blanket, tuck it tightly around the mattress so it reaches only as far as your baby's chest.

- Don't smoke around babies. Don't take babies to smoky places. Smoking during pregnancy is associated with an increased risk of SIDS.

- Avoid overheating the baby with heavy pajamas, blankets, or heaters. The bedroom temperature should be comfortable for a lightly clothed adult.

- Place the baby in her own bed to sleep. You may bring the baby into the parent's bed for nursing or comforting, but put her back in her own crib or bassinet when you are ready to go to sleep.

- Consider giving the baby a pacifier. Evidence shows that using a pacifier may reduce the risk of SIDS.

- Avoid commercial devices, including sleep positioners, that are marketed to reduce the risk of SIDS. There is no evidence that they are effective.

It is important to remember that if the baby is warm and not breathing, start CPR right away. Don't waste time. Begin chest compressions, then call EMS after about 2 minutes of CPR.

For more information, see the American Academy of Pediatrics policy statement on SIDS at http://aappolicy.aappublications.org/cgi/content/abstract/pediatrics;116/5/1245.

APPENDICES

Appendix A
Common Childhood Illnesses

● Anal Itching

Possible Causes: Pinworms, Inadequate Toilet Hygiene, Tight Underwear or Pants

What You Should Know

Pinworms are small, white, thread-like worms that live in the intestine. These parasites are about the length of a staple. The infection is spread by tiny pinworm eggs that can only be seen with a microscope. Pinworms are common among young children. Young children often do not wash their hands well and put their hands in their mouths. Many children who have pinworms do not have noticeable symptoms. Pinworms are very contagious in a family or child care setting. The pinworm eggs spread to others when a child scratches the anal area, gets eggs under the fingernails, and then touches food or other items that might be put in the mouth. It also spreads from eggs on pajamas, linens, underpants, and so on.

Pinworms can be diagnosed by collecting specimens from the anal skin. A simple test is the "Scotch tape test." Apply Scotch tape to the child's anus (rectum) first thing in the morning to collect any small, white, thread-like pinworms. Remove the tape and place another piece of tape over it to seal it. The specimen can then be taken to your medical provider or laboratory.

Poor toilet hygiene is common among young children: Girls do not wipe after urinating; boys or girls do not wipe well after a bowel movement. Skin in the area that is damp or soiled may become irritated and itch.

If clothing worn over the anal area is too small, the child may frequently clutch and pull at the clothing.

What You Should Look For

- Itching and irritation around the anal or vaginal area
- Irritated or soiled skin and underpants
- Clutching at underwear, shorts, tights, or pants

What You Should Do

Parents or primary caregiver should

 Discourage scratching of the anal area.

 Encourage your child to wash hands after using the toilet and before touching food or anything that goes into the mouth.

 Encourage girls to dry the vaginal area after urinating. Encourage both boys and girls to wipe feces off the skin after bowel movements (wiping front to back).

 Check whether underwear, tights, shorts, or pants are too small for comfort.

 If pinworms are the problem, get advice about testing and treatment from your medical provider.

 Trim the child's fingernails short.

 Wash child's bed linen, clothing, and towels in hot water. Dry in the dryer on the hottest setting. Don't shake items. This will scatter the eggs.

 Wash and sanitize toys and any surfaces that might have pinworm eggs. Some of these areas are those used for eating, toileting, hand washing, food preparation, and diapering.

Other caregivers should

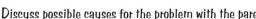 Tell the child's parents if you notice signs and symptoms of pinworms.

Discuss possible causes for the problem with the parents.

 If pinworms are the problem, watch for symptoms in others who have been exposed. Alert parents of other children who might have been exposed to watch for signs and symptoms of pinworms.

Child May Return to School or Child Care . . .

Children do not need to be kept from attending school or child care for anal itching, even if the symptoms are caused by pinworms.

Constipation

What You Should Know

Constipation is defined as hard stools that are difficult to pass. It can be caused by not drinking as much fluid as the body needs and not eating enough fiber. Sometimes it may result from postponing or resisting the urge to have a bowel movement.

What You Should Look For

- Many days without normal bowel movements
- Hard stools that are difficult or painful to pass or stools that are unusually large or hard to flush down the toilet
- Abdominal pain (stomach aches, cramping, nausea)
- Rectal bleeding from tears, called fissures
- Soiling of underwear in a child who has learned to use the toilet
- Poor appetite
- Cranky behavior

What You Should Do

Parents or primary caregiver should

 Encourage your child to drink enough clear fluids to keep the urine pale colored.

 Encourage your child to eat foods that contain fiber. These foods soften the stool. Some high-fiber foods are whole-grain products, peaches, prunes, and grapes. Other foods are raisins, plums, melons, carrots, celery, and lettuce.

 Reduce intake of foods that bind. Some foods that bind are milk, hard cheese, cottage cheese, and bananas. Other foods are apples, applesauce, and white-flour baked goods.

 Encourage going to the toilet at regular times when the child might need to have a stool. For most people, the urge to have a bowel movement comes after eating or exercising.

If your child has other caregivers, talk with them about the problem. Ask them to set regular times for the child to have a relaxed opportunity to use the toilet. Schedule times when the child is most likely to feel the urge to have a bowel movement—usually after meals or after exercise.

 Call your medical provider if the problem lasts for several weeks. Get medical care sooner if the child starts vomiting or the abdomen looks larger.

Other caregivers should

Tell parents if you think a child is constipated.

Child May Return to School or Child Care . . .

The child need not be kept from attending school or child care.

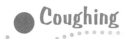 Coughing

What You Should Know

Coughing is a symptom of an irritation anywhere within the respiratory tract. Children often have a cough when they have a viral infection such as a cold. Other causes of coughing are ear infection, allergy, asthma, or croup. An infection in any part of the body involved in breathing also can cause coughing.

What You Should Look For

- Sore throat
- Dry or wet cough
- Throat irritation
- Hoarse voice, barking cough

What You Should Do

Parents or primary caregiver should

 Teach your child to "give coughs and sneezes a cold shoulder." Use the shoulder or elbow to cover the nose and mouth when having to cough or sneeze if a tissue is not handy.

 Have the child wash her hands well and often.

Watch for signs that your child is having trouble breathing. See *Chapter 3: Breathing Problems.* Always get medical care right away for a child who is having trouble breathing.

 Get medical care if your child develops a fever or if the cough lasts longer than 1 week.

Other caregivers should

 Tell parents if you notice the child is coughing.

Encourage the child to use good hygiene to avoid the spread of germs.

Call the parents or get medical care right away if the child is having trouble breathing.

Child May Return to School or Child Care . . .

The child need not be kept from attending school or child care unless the cough is severe or she is having trouble breathing.

Possible Cause: Pertussis (Whooping Cough)

What You Should Know

Pertussis is commonly known as "whooping cough." This is because of the whooping noise a child makes when coughing. It is a highly contagious bacterial infection that spreads to others through coughing and sneezing. The incubation period averages from 7 to 10 days, with a range of from 5 to 21 days. It is generally a mild illness in older children. In babies, pertussis can cause breathing problems and be life threatening.

Pertussis is diagnosed by nasal culture. It is treated with antibiotics for 5 to 14 days. A vaccine is given to babies as part of the DPT (diphtheria, pertussis, tetanus) immunization. Immunity takes several doses of vaccine. A child needs boosters to stay protected.

What You Should Look For

- Begins with cold-like signs or symptoms
- Coughing may progress to severe coughing; coughing may be so severe that it causes vomiting, loss of breath, difficulty catching breath, and blueness of lips
- Whooping sound when inhaling after a period of coughing
- The child may not have a fever or have only a slight fever

What You Should Do

Parents or primary caregiver should

 Get medical care if your child has a prolonged cough (more than 2 weeks).

2 Make sure your child gets all recommended immunizations.

3 Cases of pertussis should be reported to local health authorities.

 Watch other family members for respiratory signs or symptoms for 21 days after the child is diagnosed and begins treatment.

5 Be sure to give every dose of medicine as prescribed. Give all doses of the medicine until it is gone. Don't stop giving the medicine just because the child gets better.

Other caregivers should

 Encourage parents of a child with a prolonged cough to get medical care.

 Alert other parents if their children have been exposed to a child who is diagnosed with pertussis. Encourage them to call their medical providers. Keep the identity of the sick child confidential.

3 Monitor others who might have been exposed to the child for respiratory problems. If a persistent cough develops, they should get medical care.

Child May Return to School or Child Care ...

The child may return to school or child care after 5 days on antibiotic therapy. This medicine must be continued for the total number of days prescribed. Depending on the antibiotic used, the total treatment time can be 5–14 days.

Diaper Rash

Possible Cause: Simple Diaper Rash

What You Should Know

Diaper rash commonly occurs when surfaces that are wet by urine or stool rub against the skin. Also, bacteria in the bowel react with urine to form ammonia. This may irritate the skin. Diaper rash can be painful.

What You Should Look For

- Redness
- Raw skin
- Red bumps
- Sores
- Cracking of skin in the diaper region

What You Should Do

Parents or primary caregiver should

 1. Keep the child as dry as possible. One way is to use commercially available disposable diapers that are designed to keep moisture away from the skin.

2. Change diapers often. Check your child's diaper every hour: look, feel, and smell the diaper through the clothing. At least every 2 hours, open the diaper to look for wetness or stool.

3. Wash diaper area with soap and warm water; allow to dry completely.

 4. Place child in cool baths with one-half cup vinegar for 15 to 20 minutes several times per day. Vinegar reduces bacterial growth. It helps to neutralize ammonia.

 5. Protect diaper area with over-the-counter ointments. Examples are zinc oxide or petroleum jelly. These act as moisture barriers.

 6. Wash hands well after removing soiled diapers and clothing. It is important to wash your hands even if you wore gloves during the changing.

7. Do not use baby powder or cornstarch. These are not recommended.

8. If you are using cloth diapers, they should have an absorbent inner lining completely contained within an outer covering of waterproof material. The outer covering and inner lining are changed together as a unit. Remove the liner and diaper when soiled. Then it should be cleaned, disinfected, washed, rinsed, and dried or chemically disinfected. Rinsing in a dilute solution of vinegar may help remove any detergent that was left behind. Rinsing also helps remove any other chemicals that might irritate the child's skin.

Other caregivers should

Tell parents if you notice that the child has a diaper rash.

Child May Return to School or Child Care . . .

The child need not be kept from attending school or child care.

Possible Cause: Candida Diaper Infection

What You Should Know

Candida is a type of yeast that lives in the intestines of healthy people. It can infect moist areas of skin. It is treated with prescription medicine. To learn more, see the section on "Thrush."

What You Should Look For

• A fiery red rash

What You Should Do

Parents or primary caregiver should

 Talk to your medical provider about the rash. She may prescribe a medicated cream.

 Change diapers often. Sanitize the diaper changing area after each diaper change.

 Clean the skin in the diaper area carefully. Dry the area completely.

 Apply a thin layer of any cream that has been prescribed to the affected skin.

 Wash hands well after each diaper change.

Other caregivers should

 Wash and sanitize diaper changing areas after each diaper change.

 Keep the child's skin clean and dry.

 Talk to parents about the rash.

Child May Return to School or Child Care . . .

The child need not be kept from attending school or daycare.

Diarrhea

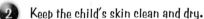

What You Should Know

Diarrhea is watery stool. They are less formed than usual and more frequent. Diarrhea is caused mostly by viruses. Sometimes it can be caused by bacterial or parasitic infections. Some medicines (especially antibiotics), changes in diet, and certain foods also can cause diarrhea. It may resolve without treatment within a few days. If mild diarrhea does not resolve within a few days or if there is blood in the diarrhea, get medical care. Your medical provider may want to do a stool culture to see if the diarrhea is infectious.

What You Should Look For

- Frequent, loose or watery stools compared with the child's normal pattern
- Abdominal cramps
- Fever
- Generally not feeling well
- Blood in the stool

What You Should Do

Parents or primary caregiver should

 Do not let children and adults who have diarrhea handle food.

 Be very careful about good hygiene. Wash hands well and often, especially after using the toilet or handling soiled diapers. Always wash hands before anything having to do with food preparation or eating.

Get medical care if your child has any of the following:
- ► Blood in stool
- ► Frequent vomiting
- ► Abdominal pain
- ► Less frequent urination
- ► No tears when crying
- ► Loss of appetite for liquids
- ► High fever
- ► Frequent or persistent diarrhea
- ► Dry, sticky mouth
- ► Weight loss
- ► Extreme thirst

 Don't take a child in diapers to a child care facility if he has diarrhea. This also applies to children who use the toilet but are having "accidents" because of diarrhea.

Other caregivers should

 Tell parents if a child has diarrhea.

Be very careful about good hygiene. Wash hands well and often, especially after using the toilet or handling soiled diapers. Always wash hands before anything having to do with food preparation or eating.

 Ask parents not to bring a child in diapers if the child has diarrhea. This also applies to children who use the toilet but are having "accidents" because of diarrhea.

Child May Return to School or Child Care . . .

- The child needs approval by a medical provider to return if the diarrhea was caused by certain bacteria. Examples are shigella, salmonella, and some types of E. coli. A child whose diarrhea was caused by the parasite *Giardia lamblia* also needs approval.

- A toilet-trained child may return when the stool can be contained in the toilet.

- Even if stools stay loose, the child may return when he seems well and the stool consistency has not changed for a week. If your child needs special care, the staff should decide if they can provide the care while still taking care of the other children in the group.

Possible Cause: *Escherichia coli* diarrhea

What You Should Know

Many types of E. coli bacteria live normally in the intestine; however, at least five types are known to cause diarrhea. Two types have caused many outbreaks in group care settings. Infections with a certain type of E. coli may cause other severe problems. One severe problem is bleeding from irritation of the bowel. Other severe problems are kidney damage and blood cell damage. The incubation period ranges from 1 to 8 days. The child is contagious until the diarrhea goes away and test results come back negative twice.

One way E. coli is spread is through direct contact with infected people. Another way is by drinking contaminated water, such as untreated drinking water in recreation areas and in some foreign countries. These bacteria also are spread by eating contaminated food. Examples are undercooked ground beef and unpasteurized milk and yogurt. Other foods that have caused E. coli are apple cider, raw vegetables, and salami. Some E. coli problems can be prevented by cooking all ground beef so there is no pink meat and only using pasteurized products.

What You Should Look For

- Loose stools, which may be watery and bloody
- Abdominal pain
- Fever

What You Should Do

Parents or primary caregiver should

 Get medical care if your child has signs and symptoms of *E. coli*.

 Wash hands often, especially before preparing food.

 Make sure any ground beef your child eats is cooked well done. Use only pasteurized products.

 Don't let your child drink untreated water.

Other caregivers should

 Tell parents if a child has *E. coli* symptoms.

 Wear disposable gloves when changing diaper or helping with toileting. This will reduce the spread of infections. Wash hands well after removing gloves.

 Practice good hygiene. Wash hands often, especially before preparing food.

 Understand ways that *E. coli* is spread. Avoid giving children foods that are known to spread the bacteria. Don't let children drink untreated water.

Child May Return to School or Child Care . . .

When your medical provider gives approval.

Possible Cause: Infectious Diarrhea

What You Should Know

Infectious diarrhea varies from mild to severe. It is highly contagious. The disease is spread through contaminated water or food. It is caused by viruses or bacteria. Salmonella and shigella are two types of bacteria that can cause it. Infectious diarrhea also can be caused by a parasite, such as *Giardia lamblia*. Some causes can be diagnosed by stool culture. Bacterial infections are treated with prescription medicine. Other types of infection do not respond to medicine. The body has to rid itself of these types of infections.

What You Should Look For

- Diarrhea containing blood or mucus
- Stomach or abdominal cramping and gas
- Foul-smelling stools
- Fever
- Weight loss

What You Should Do

Parents or primary caregiver should

 Contact your medical provider to learn what to do for treatment. Also find out how to prevent spread of the disease to other family members.

 Encourage your child to drink extra amounts of clear fluids, but not fruit juices.

Do not allow your child to share drinking glasses or eating utensils with others.

Other caregivers should

 Wear disposable gloves when changing diapers or helping with toileting. This will reduce chances of spreading infection. Wash hands well after removing gloves.

Report symptoms of infectious diarrhea to parents.

Child May Return to School or Child Care . . .

- When treatment and any required laboratory tests have been completed. *Note:* Salmonella is not always treated with medicine. Children who have no symptoms but have *Giardia lamblia* in their stools do not need to be kept from attending school or child care.
- In all cases, check with your medical provider if your child has tested positive for infectious diarrhea.

Possible Cause: Hepatitis A

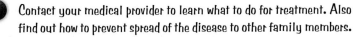

What You Should Know

Hepatitis A is a viral infection. It causes inflammation of the liver. The virus is spread from person to person when hands contaminated with microscopic particles of stool touch food or eating utensils. Infected children do not always have symptoms. Infected adults, however, can be very sick. People who have the infection are most contagious for 2 weeks before signs or symptoms develop. The infection can be in the incubation (developing) stage for 1 to 2 months before there are any symptoms. Those who have hepatitis A are not contagious after about a week after the jaundice develops.

What You Should Look For

- Fever
- Jaundice (yellowing of skin or whites of eyes)
- Abdominal discomfort
- Tiredness
- Dark-brown urine
- Loss of appetite
- Nausea

What You Should Do

Parents or primary caregiver should

 Prevent the disease by getting the hepatitis A vaccine.

 If anyone in your family is exposed to someone with hepatitis A, get medical care right away. If you think that you or a family member might have the disease, get medical care right away.

 Do not allow your child to share drinking glasses or eating utensils with others.

Other caregivers should

Wear disposable gloves when changing diapers or helping with toileting. This will help reduce chances of spreading infection. Remove gloves *after* disposing of soiled clothing and *before* putting on clean undergarments. Wipe hands with a disposable wipe immediately after removing gloves. Then wash hands well as the last step in the diapering or toileting process.

Inform parents if you notice symptoms of the disease.

Contact your medical provider if you are exposed to the hepatitis A virus.

Child May Return to School or Child Care . . .

- Child should remain at home for 1 week after developing symptoms.
- Check with your medical provider about protection of others who may have been exposed to hepatitis A infection.

Possible Cause: Rotavirus

What You Should Know

Rotavirus is a virus that belongs to a family of viruses found worldwide. It is one of the most common causes of diarrhea and vomiting, especially from late fall to early spring. It is the single most common cause of diarrhea in children younger than 2 years. Rotavirus can cause serious illness in babies and toddlers. Nearly all children have been infected with it by age 3 years. Children can become infected more than once because the virus has many types. It is spread from person to person when hands contaminated with microscopic particles of stool touch food or eating utensils. The incubation period is from 2 to 4 days. The child is contagious up to 3 weeks after the illness.

What You Should Look For

- Nonbloody diarrhea
- Nausea
- Vomiting
- Dehydration in severe cases
- Generally lasts from 3 to 8 days

What You Should Do

Parents or primary caregiver should

 Always practice proper hand washing. This is very important after changing diapers or toileting. It also is very important before any contact with food or surfaces involved in preparing and serving food.

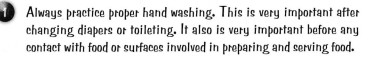 Practice proper cleaning and sanitizing of surfaces. After surfaces are visibly clean, apply a sanitizer solution. Leave it in contact with the surface for the time recommended on the product label. See "How to Clean Up Body Fluids to Prevent the Spread of Germs" in **Chapter 4.**

Make an extra effort to practice frequent and correct hand washing, as well as cleaning and sanitizing of surfaces if your child has the virus.

Talk with your medical provider about the rotavirus vaccine.

Other caregivers should

 Alert parents when an outbreak occurs so they can watch for symptoms.

Make an extra effort to practice frequent and correct hand washing, as well as cleaning and sanitizing of surfaces, whenever an outbreak occurs.

 Educate parents about how to prevent the spread of this illness in their families. Make them aware that there is a vaccine to protect children from rotavirus.

Child May Return to School or Child Care . . .

A toilet-trained child may return when the stool can be contained in the toilet. For a child using diapers, he may return when he seems well and the stool consistency has not changed for a week. If your child needs special care, the staff should decide if they can provide the care while still taking care of the other children in the group.

Possible Cause: Shigella

What You Should Know

Shigella is an infection caused by the shigella bacteria. The virus is spread from person to person when hands contaminated with microscopic particles of stool touch food or eating utensils. Children younger than 5 years, adults who care for young children, and others living in crowded conditions are at increased risk. The incubation period is from 1 to 7 days. If left untreated, shigella bacteria can live in the stool of an infected person for up to 4 weeks.

What You Should Look For

- Loose, watery stools with blood or mucus
- Fever
- Headache
- Convulsions
- Abdominal pain

What You Should Do

Parents or primary caregiver should

 Always practice proper hand washing. This is very important after changing diapers or toileting. It also is very important before any contact with food or surfaces involved in preparing and serving food.

 Contact your medical provider if your child has symptoms.

Do not allow your child to share water play areas where water from a clean water source is not free flowing. An example is a water table with one large bin into which many children put their hands.

Other caregivers should

 Alert parents if their child has symptoms or if other children at the facility have diarrhea.

 Be sure everyone with diarrhea is tested. Notify the health department so that arrangements can be made to test the stool of everyone who has diarrhea.

 Stop food handling or feeding of others by individuals with diarrhea.

Arrange for grouping together of children and adults who are well but still have positive stool tests for shigella.

Child May Return to School or Child Care . . .

When treatment is complete and test results from stool cultures are negative.

Ear Pain

Possible Cause: Otitis Media (Middle Ear Infection)

What You Should Know

A middle ear infection most often occurs when mucus builds up in the middle ear space. The mucus can come from a cold or allergy. It also can come from something that irritates the respiratory system. Mucus collects more easily in small children. This is because the eustachian tube that normally drains the middle ear is small and easily blocked. Most middle ear infections are caused by viruses. They resolve themselves in a day or two and are not contagious.

What You Should Look For

- Fever
- Pain or irritability
- Difficulty hearing
- Blocked ears

- Drainage
- Swelling around ear

What You Should Do

Parents or primary caregiver should

 Make sure a child with a respiratory infection drinks plenty of fluids.

 Prevent room air from becoming too dry. Dry air tends to dry out the secretions. This makes them thicker and harder to drain.

 Ventilate indoor spaces with fresh outdoor air at least daily. This will help to reduce the number of germs in the air.

 Follow your medical provider's instructions to take care of the ear infection. Find out what to do if your child has ear pain.

 Do not allow your child to drink from a bottle while lying on his back. This position lets fluid enter the eustachian tube. The fluid causes irritation, which can make it easier for an ear infection to start.

Watch for hearing loss or speech problems in a child who gets ear infections one after another.

Other caregivers should

Tell parents if you notice a child has signs and symptoms of an ear infection.

Child May Return to School or Child Care . . .

The child may return when he feels well enough to do regular activities. If your child needs special care, the staff should decide if they can provide the care while still taking care of the other children in the group.

Eye Irritation/Pain

Possible Cause: Conjunctivitis (Pink Eye)

What You Should Know

Pink eye is an inflammation of the thin tissue covering the white part of the eye and the inside of the eyelids. (Inflammation is redness and swelling.) There are several types of pink eye. Some types are bacterial, viral, allergic, and chemical. The infectious type is easily spread. If a child touches discharge from an infected eye on a surface and then touches her own eye area, she can get pink eye.

What You Should Look For

- Red, irritated, or painful eye(s)
- Yellow or watery drainage
- Eyelids temporarily stuck together from encrusted discharge when child wakes up from sleep
- Watery drainage is most likely viral pink eye, a sign of allergy or chemical irritation
- Green or yellow drainage (pus) is most likely bacterial pink eye; it may be treated with an antibiotic

What You Should Do

Parents or primary caregiver should

 Clean drainage from child's eye(s) as needed. Use a clean tissue or gauze pad and warm water. Wipe each eye outward from inner corner (from nose to ear).

2 Try to keep the child from touching her eye(s).

3 Wash your hands well. Encourage your child to do the same.

4 Contact your medical provider to find out if your child needs medical care.

5 Apply antibiotic drops or ointment if prescribed.

Other caregivers should

 Tell parents if you notice a child with signs and symptoms of pink eye. A child with irritated eyes needs to see a medical provider.

 Contact the health department about how to keep infectious pink eye from spreading.

Child May Return to School or Child Care . . .

- Generally, children do not need to be kept from attending school or child care unless their eyes are red and they have green or yellow drainage (pus). This suggests the possibility of bacterial infection. If this is the problem, the child may return after she starts treatment with an antibiotic.
- The child may return when she feels well enough to do regular activities. If your child needs special care, the staff should decide if they can provide the care while still taking care of the other children in the group.

Possible Cause: Sty

What You Should Know

A sty is an infection of an oil gland inside the eyelid that creates a swelling. The swelling is usually near the eyelashes.

What You Should Look For

A lump in the eyelid, which may or may not be painful

What You Should Do

Parents or primary caregiver should

 Apply a warm wash cloth to the eye as often and for as long as possible during the day.

 Try to keep the child from touching her eye(s).

3 Wash your hands well. Encourage your child to do the same.

4 Call your medical provider if the sty doesn't improve.

Other caregivers should

Tell parents if you notice a child has signs and symptoms of a sty.

Child May Return to School or Child Care . . .

The child need not be kept from attending school or child care for a sty.

 Fever

Possible Causes: Infection, Overheating, or Reaction to a Medicine

What You Should Know

Fever alone is not harmful. When a child has an infection, the body's normal defense is to raise the body temperature. In young children a rapid rise of body temperature may sometimes cause a febrile seizure. This type of seizure is usually outgrown by 6 years of age. Fever is not a reason to send a child home from school. It is a reason to check for a cause of the fever. It also is a reason to monitor the child for other symptoms of illness.

What You Should Look For

- Flushed skin
- Tiredness
- Irritability
- Decreased activity
- 100° F axillary (armpit)
- 101° F orally
- 102° F rectally
- Temperature taken with a tool that is used in the child's ear or against the child's temple gives a reading that is the same as an oral or rectal temperature reading

What You Should Do

Parents or primary caregiver should

 Do not give aspirin. Give fever-reducing medicine if your medical provider has told you to.

 Try to figure out the cause of the fever. Give first aid care for the cause. For example, if your child is overheated, cool him off. Perhaps the cause is a recent vaccine or medicine. If your child is acting sick, follow the Six Steps of Pediatric First Aid.

 Get medical care as soon as possible for a baby younger than 4 months with an unexplained temperature of 100° F axillary (armpit) or 101° F rectally or higher. Any baby younger than 2 months with a temperature this high should get medical care within an hour.

Other caregivers should

Tell parents if a child has a fever.

Child May Return to School or Child Care . . .

Fever is not a reason to keep a child from attending school or child care.

 Headache

What You Should Know

Most headaches are minor and are caused by overexertion or stress. A headache might be a sign of the beginning of illness. It also might be a sign of a vision problem.

What You Should Look For

- Tiredness and irritability
- Head holding

What You Should Do

Parents or primary caregiver should

 Have your child rest in a quiet, darkened area.

 Give any medicine prescribed by the child's medical provider.

 Contact your medical provider if the child has a sudden, severe headache with vomiting. Contact your medical provider if your child has a stiff neck that keeps him from putting his chin down when asked to "look at your belly button." These symptoms might be a sign of a life-threatening infection called meningitis.

 Discuss your child's headaches with your medical provider if they are severe or if your child gets them often.

Other caregivers should

Tell parents if their child is having frequent headaches.

Child May Return to School or Child Care . . .

A headache is not a reason to keep a child from attending school or child care. The child may return when he feels well enough to do regular activities. If your child needs special care, the staff should decide if they can provide the care while still taking care of the other children in the group.

Influenza

Possible Cause: Influenza Virus

What You Should Know

Influenza (the flu) is a contagious disease. It is caused by a group of respiratory viruses called the influenza viruses. The flu is spread through direct contact from sneezing and coughing. The contagious period lasts from the day before signs or symptoms appear until 7 days after the onset of flu.

What You Should Look For

- Sudden onset of fever
- Headache
- Chills
- Muscle aches and pains
- Sore throat
- Cough
- Mild pink eye
- Decreased energy
- Abdominal pain
- Nausea and vomiting

What You Should Do

Parents or primary caregiver should

 Practice careful and frequent hand washing after any contact with surfaces that might have nasal secretions on them.

 Teach children to wash their hands after sneezing, coughing, or using a tissue.

 Teach your child to "give coughs and sneezes a cold shoulder." Use the shoulder or elbow to cover the nose and mouth when having to cough or sneeze if a tissue is not handy.

 Avoid using any product that contains aspirin.

Other caregivers should

 Everyone involved in child care should get the flu vaccine.

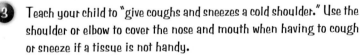 Take steps to limit the spread of germs.

Tell parents if you notice a child has signs and symptoms of the flu. Also make parents aware of a flu outbreak in the facility.

Child May Return to School or Child Care . . .

When symptoms resolve. The child need not be kept from attending school or child care. The child may return when he feels well enough to do regular activities. If your child needs special care, the staff should decide if they can provide the care while still taking care of the other children in the group.

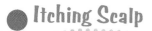

Itching Scalp

Possible Cause: Head Lice

What You Should Know

Head lice are tiny insects that live on the scalp and hair. They are diagnosed by finding tiny yellow/white eggs, called nits. Nits can be found firmly attached to a shaft of hair. Nits can be found all along hair shafts and all over the head. Good places to look for nits are at the crown, the nape of the neck, and behind the ears. Adult lice are harder to find.

Lice are spread from person to person by crawling. A child can get lice by sharing personal items, such as hats, combs, and brushes. Lice cannot jump or fly. They are not carried by cats or dogs. Lice are not caused by poor hygiene.

All family members who have lice must be treated at the same time. The safest and most effective way to get rid of head lice is with a special lice comb. Finding and combing out all of the nits and lice is very tedious. Lice-killing shampoos are available. They are pesticides. Use them carefully. Follow the manufacturer's instructions. Household remedies do not work.

What You Should Look For

- Persistent itching on scalp
- Tiny red bites on scalp and on hairline
- Open sores and crusting

What You Should Do

Parents or primary caregiver should

 Treat with lice-killing shampoo as recommended by child's medical provider. Follow package directions. Wear disposable gloves when applying shampoo.

 Do not repeat treatment unless the product directions tell you to apply it more than once. Even then, do not repeat it without asking a medical provider. Often dandruff can be mistaken for nits. Old, empty nits (eggs) may be present. These aren't a problem.

 Scrub hair brushes, combs, and hair accessories. Then soak them in very hot water for 10 minutes.

Treat all family members who have lice at the same time.

 Remove all nits and live lice with a small nit comb or with fingernails. Nit combs are available in pharmacies.

 Check all family members' heads daily for 10 days.

 Clean bed linens, blankets, towels, clothing, jackets, and hats. Machine wash all washable items in hot water. Dry them in the dryer on the hottest setting. Send other items out to be dry-cleaned.

 Place pillows and stuffed animals in dryer on hot setting for 30 minutes.

 Place items that cannot be washed or dried in a closed plastic bag for 2 weeks.

 Vacuum upholstered furniture, mattresses, rugs, car seats, and stuffed toys.

 Do not use lice sprays.

Other caregivers should

 Tell parents if you notice a child has signs and symptoms of lice.

 Notify all parents of a case of lice. Keep the name of the infected child confidential.

 Clean items that may have been infected as described in the section for parents and primary caregiver.

Child May Return to School or Child Care . . .

- The child does not have to be kept from attending school or child care before the end of the day on which the lice is discovered.
- The child may return after treatment with lice-killing shampoo and thorough nit removal.

● Lyme Disease

What You Should Know

Lyme disease is an infection that is spread by deer ticks. When the tick bites and feeds, it deposits the waste from its gut into the wound where it is feeding. This infects the wound with a type of bacteria known as spirochetes. Lyme disease is not contagious.

The incubation period is from 3 to 31 days from the tick bite until a rash appears. Lyme disease can be controlled by avoiding places where deer ticks live. If bitten by a tick, quickly removing the tick will lessen the chance of getting the disease.

What You Should Look For

- A large, circular, or oval-shaped rash that appears after a tick bite; in the center will be a partial clear area; the rash gradually gets bigger
- Fever
- Headache
- Mild neck stiffness
- Flulike signs or symptoms
- Untreated Lyme disease may lead to arthritis, neurologic problems, cardiac problems, or meningitis

What You Should Do

Parents or primary caregiver should

 Avoid places where deer ticks live.

 If the child will be in an area where deer ticks live, use protection. Apply permethrin to clothing or DEET to skin. You cannot use permethrin or DEET on babies younger than 2 months. Use DEET only between 10% and 30%. DEET solutions of 10% are effective for about 2 hours. Lower concentrations are effective for shorter periods of time.

3 Inspect your child's skin and scalp after possible tick exposure.

4 Remove any ticks found on the child with tweezers. See "First Aid Care for Tick Bites" in *Chapter 9: Bites and Stings*. Remove a tick carefully. You want to avoid rupturing the tick. This will cause more infection to get into the wound.

 Get medical care if your child gets a rash after a tick bite.

Other caregivers should

Inform parents if you find a tick on a child.

Child May Return to School or Child Care . . .

The child need not be kept from attending school or child care.

Measles

What You Should Know

Measles is a viral disease caused by the measles virus. It is highly contagious. Although there is a vaccine, outbreaks continue to occur among those who have not been protected by the vaccine. It is spread by droplets from sneezing and coughing. The measles are contagious from 1 to 2 days before the first signs or symptoms appear (usually from 3 to 5 days before the rash) until 4 days after the rash appears.

What You Should Look For

- Fever, cough, runny nose, and red, watery eyes
- Small red spots in mouth
- Appearance of rash at the hairline spreading downward over the body
- May have diarrhea or ear infection
- Complications may be serious; some are pneumonia, brain inflammation, and convulsions; deafness and mental retardation are others

What You Should Do

Parents or primary caregiver should

 Keep your child's vaccines up-to-date. Make sure everyone in your family is protected from the measles. Everyone needs two doses of MMR vaccine unless they were born before 1957.

 Get medical care if your child becomes infected with measles.

Other caregivers should

 Make sure all adults and children at the facility have been immunized. Everyone needs two doses of MMR vaccine unless they were born before 1957. Review all immunization records.

 Practice proper hand washing.

 Practice routine infection control measures.

Tell parents if you notice a child has signs and symptoms of the measles. Also make parents aware of a measles outbreak in the facility.

5 Report the infection to the health department.

6 Any children who might be exposed to the infection and who have weakened immune systems should not attend school or child care. This also includes those who haven't been vaccinated. These children must not attend for 2 weeks after the last child breaks out in the measles rash.

Child May Return to School or Child Care . . .

- Four days after the beginning of the rash.
- The child may return when he feels well enough to do regular activities. If your child needs special care, the staff should decide if they can provide the care while still taking care of the other children in the group.

Mouth/Lip Sores

Possible Cause: Herpes Simplex Virus

What You Should Know

Herpes simplex virus is a viral disease. It causes a variety of infections in different age groups. It is usually painful. Once someone is infected, the virus can become active again from time to time. In children it usually appears as a sore near the mouth or nose ("cold sore") or in the mouth. The child is contagious until the sore is dry (on the lip or nose) or goes away (in the mouth).

This virus is spread by direct contact with the sore. It also is spread by secretions from the sore that get on other surfaces, such as toys. A child who has mouth ulcers and blisters and does not have control of drooling should not be in a child care setting. Anyone who has a sore on some other body area that cannot be completely covered should not be in a child care setting.

What You Should Look For

- Painful, small, fluid-filled blisters in the mouth, on gums, or on lips
- Blisters that weep clear fluid and are slow to crust over
- Irritability
- Fever
- Tender, swollen lymph nodes

What You Should Do

Parents or primary caregiver should

 Contact your medical provider to find out what to do.

 Keep area of sores clean and dry.

 Try to keep child from touching an open cold sore.

 Be very careful about good hygiene. Wash hands well whenever you might have touched something that was infected. Wash hands well and often, especially after using the toilet or handling soiled diapers. Always wash hands before anything having to do with food preparation or eating.

 Wash and sanitize toys that the child puts in her mouth. Also sanitize bottle nipples and utensils that have come into contact with saliva. Wash and sanitize items that have been touched by children who are drooling and put fingers in their mouths.

Other caregivers should

 Alert parents if you notice symptoms in a child.

 If a child does have the virus, inform other parents, family members, and staff who may have been exposed so they can watch for symptoms.

 Make sure everyone on staff practices good hygiene.

Child May Return to School or Child Care . . .

- When an open sore has completely scabbed over or can be completely covered. Also when a child who has mouth sores and blisters is not drooling.
- The child may return when she feels well enough to do regular activities. If your child needs special care, the staff should decide if they can provide the care while still taking care of the other children in the group.

Possible Cause: Hand, Foot, and Mouth Syndrome
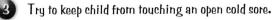

What You Should Know

Hand, foot, and mouth syndrome is a common viral infection. It is usually mild and occurs more often in the summer and fall. Young children are more likely than older children or adults to get the disease. Common signs are blisters in the child's mouth and on the palms and soles of the feet. Fever is another common sign. The infection is spread from person to person through respiratory secretions and stool. The incubation period is from 3 to 6 days. The illness usually resolves on its own in about 1 week. The virus can be present in stool for several weeks after infection starts. It can be spread by people who have no symptoms.

What You Should Look For

- Tiny blisters or ulcers in the mouth and blisters on the fingers, palms of hands, and the soles of feet

- May see common cold signs or symptoms with fever, sore throat, runny nose, and cough

- Blisters in the mouth that make it difficult for the child to eat or drink

- Other signs or symptoms, such as vomiting and diarrhea

What You Should Do

Parents or primary caregiver should

 Get medical care if your child seems very sick or uncomfortable.

 Don't break blisters. They heal better if not broken.

 Encourage your child to drink small amounts often. This will prevent dehydration.

Other caregivers should

 Tell parents if you notice a child has signs and symptoms of hand, foot, and mouth syndrome. Encourage parents to get medical care if the child seems very sick or uncomfortable.

 Practice good hand-washing routines, especially after toileting or diaper changing.

Child May Return to School or Child Care ...

The child need not be kept from attending school or child care. The child may return when he feels well enough to do regular activities. If your child needs special care, the staff should decide if they can provide the care while still taking care of the other children in the group. *Note:* Exclusion will not reduce spread of the disease. This is because some children may not know they have the disease and still be contagious. The virus is also present for weeks in the stool after the child's symptoms are gone.

Possible Cause: Thrush

What You Should Know

Thrush is a yeast infection in the mouth. It seldom occurs in children older than 6 months. The fungus is widespread in the environment. It can be found especially in warm and moist tissues. The fungus causes disease when it outgrows healthy germs in the lining of the mouth. This infection is usually treated with antifungal medicine.

What You Should Look For

- White patches on the inside of cheeks and on gums and tongue

What You Should Do

Parents or primary caregiver should

 Talk to your medical provider about the disease. Follow instructions for medicine and other treatment. The goal is to reduce the amount of yeast to levels that do not cause illness.

 Practice good hand-washing routines.

 Carefully wash and sanitize all items that might reinfect the child. Some examples are nipples, pacifiers, and toys that the child puts in his mouth.

Other caregivers should

 Tell parents if you notice a child has signs of thrush.

 Practice good hand-washing routines.

Do not allow babies to share toys that they put in their mouths. Wash and sanitize pacifiers or bottles between uses.

Child May Return to School or Child Care . . .

Children with thrush do not need to be kept from attending school or child care.

Skin Eruptions and Rashes

Possible Cause: Chicken Pox

What You Should Know

Chicken pox is a common viral illness lasting about 1 week. It is highly contagious. Breathing the same air as an infected person spreads the virus. It also can be spread by contact with body fluids from an infected person. The incubation period is approximately 14 to 16 days. This period can be as short as 10 days and as long as 21 days after contact. It is most contagious from 1 to 2 days before the rash appears until all the blisters have scabs and no new blisters are forming. A vaccine is recommended for everyone who has not already had chicken pox. The chicken pox virus can cause shingles. It stays alive in the body but remains inactive. Then from time to time throughout life the virus can become active again and result in shingles.

What You Should Look For

- Rash of red bumps that are filled with fluid and can break, weep, and scab; they appear primarily on the face and trunk
- Rash can also be on arms, legs, or any mucous membrane surface, such as inside the mouth, throat, eyes, and vagina
- Fever
- Runny nose
- Cough
- Itching

What You Should Do

Parents or primary caregiver should

 Avoid products that contain aspirin or aspirin-like chemicals (salicylates).

 Follow the advice of your medical provider for managing symptoms. She may recommend the use of acetaminophen for fever.

 Watch for chicken pox to develop in other family members or playmates for 3 weeks.

 Encourage your child to drink clear fluids.

Bathe your child in cool water to relieve itching. This will also help prevent secondary infection from scratching.

 Some children may be more comfortable if their itchy spots are painted with a thin film of calamine lotion. Letting a child paint her own itchy spots may be comforting.

 Trim your child's fingernails or put mittens on a baby to prevent scratching. Scratching can infect open lesions. This can lead to scarring.

 Consult your medical provider if the child seems very uncomfortable or ill.

 Be sure all family members who have not already had chicken pox and who are older than 12 months get the vaccine as quickly as possible.

Other caregivers should

 Tell parents if you notice a child has signs and symptoms of the chicken pox. Also make parents aware of a chicken pox outbreak in the facility.

 Notify health authorities when a case occurs in group care so outbreak measures can be started.

 Check immunization records for all people older than 12 months who are involved in any way with child care. Each person should be immunized.

 Be sure that anyone who has shingles covers blisters to keep the virus from spreading.

Child May Return to School or Child Care . . .
When all blisters have crusted, about 7 days.

Possible Cause: Fifth Disease
What You Should Know
Fifth disease is a mild viral illness caused by Pinworms B19. It is harmless for most children. The rash usually appears 1 to 3 weeks after the infection. The incubation period is from 4 to 14 days but may last up to 21 days. A child is contagious until the rash appears. The virus spreads through contact with throat and mouth secretions. It also spreads by exposure to blood that contains the virus. Fifth disease can be serious for an unborn child

or for children with some chronic illnesses. Examples are sickle cell anemia and thalassemia. Fifth disease also can be serious for children with suppressed immune systems, such as leukemia and AIDS patients. One bout of infection is believed to give lifelong immunity. About half of all adults have already had the disease. By the time adults reach old age, 90% have had it.

What You Should Look For

- Fever
- Muscle aches
- Joint pain
- Headache
- Red "slapped-cheek" rash
- Lacelike rash

What You Should Do

Parents or primary caregiver should

 Get medical care if your child has a chronic illness that makes him more vulnerable to infection.

 Talk to your medical provider. Find out what to do to care for your child's symptoms.

 A pregnant woman who is exposed to fifth disease should consult her medical provider. She may need a blood test to see if her baby is at risk.

Other caregivers should

 Notify parents and staff that fifth disease is common in childhood. Inform them that hand washing is the best protection from infection.

 Alert staff and parents of possible health risks to unborn babies and children with chronic illnesses.

Child May Return to School or Child Care . . .

The child need not be kept from attending school or child care unless he has a chronic illness or a compromised immune system. Children without these problems may return when they feel well enough to do regular activities. If your child needs special care, the staff should decide if they can provide the care while still taking care of the other children in the group.

Possible Cause: Heat Rash (Prickly Heat)

What You Should Know

Prickly heat is seen most often in babies and young children. It occurs during hot and humid weather. It is caused when the sweat gland openings become blocked. This results in little red bumps around the sweat duct openings.

What You Should Look For

- Tiny red bumps in areas that tend to be moist
- Commonly seen in skin folds of the neck and on the upper chest, arms, legs, and diaper area

What You Should Do

Parents or primary caregiver should

 Dress the child in clothing that keeps the skin cool and dry.

2 Pay special attention to skin folds that stay wet with perspiration, urine, or drool.

3 Use cool water to remove body oil and sweat. Then dry the area.

4 Leave areas open to air without clothing.

5 Use air conditioning or a fan blowing gently on your child to keep her cool.

6 Do not apply skin ointments.

Other caregivers should

1 Tell parents if you notice a child has signs of prickly heat.

2 Try to keep the child cool.

3 Pay attention to moist areas. Wash with cool water. Keep these areas dry.

Child May Return to School or Child Care . . .

The child need not be kept from attending school or child care.

Possible Cause: Impetigo

What You Should Know

Impetigo is a bacterial skin infection. It can develop in any skin injury, such as an insect bite, cut, or break in the skin. It can develop as a result of irritation caused by a runny nose. A child can spread the infection to other parts of his body by scratching. He can spread the germs to others in close contact by directly touching them. He can spread the germs by touching a surface that another child touches. Impetigo can occur anytime. It is most common in warm weather when cuts and scrapes from outdoor play are more likely.

What You Should Look For

- Red pimples
- Fluid-filled blisters
- Oozing rash covered by crusted yellow scabs

What You Should Do

Parents or primary caregiver should

 Call child's medical provider for a treatment plan.

 Clean infected area with soap and water. Try to gently remove crusty scabs.

Cover infected area loosely. The scabs need airflow for healing. Covering also helps prevent contact that would spread the infection to others or to other parts of the child's body.

Keep sores covered until they are healed.

Wash hands well after treating sores.

Try to keep your child from scratching.

Trim the child's fingernails.

Do not permit sharing of towels or face cloths.

Observe the rash. Notice whether it improves or gets worse.

Other caregivers should

Tell parents if you notice a child has signs of impetigo.

If the child cannot be picked up promptly, wash the affected area with soap and water. Then cover any exposed sores until the parents can arrange to remove the child for treatment.

In the event that more than one child in a group has been infected, contact the health department about control measures. The problem could involve antibiotic-resistant staphylococcal bacteria.

Child May Return to School or Child Care . . .

- Twenty-four hours after treatment is started with an antibiotic ointment or oral antibiotic medicine.

- The child may return when he feels well enough to do regular activities. If your child needs special care, the staff should decide if they can provide the care while still taking care of the other children in the group.

Possible Cause: Ringworm

What You Should Know

Ringworm is a fungal infection that can affect the body, feet, or scalp. It is mildly contagious. Symptoms vary according to the area of the body infected. Ringworm spreads from person to person by direct contact. It is spread by sharing combs, brushes, hats, hair ornaments, towels, clothing, or bedding. It is also spread by contact with infected people. Another way it is spread is by surfaces contaminated by people who have a ringworm lesion. Skin infections are treated with an antifungal topical cream. Scalp infections need an oral medicine that must be taken for weeks. The child is no longer contagious once treatment is started.

What You Should Look For

- On the body, arms, and legs: red, circular patches with raised edges and a clear area in the center
- On the feet: cracking and peeling of skin between toes
- On the scalp: itchy areas of dandruff-like scaling with or without hair loss; redness and scaling of scalp with broken hairs or patches of hair loss

What You Should Do

Parents or primary caregiver should

 Call your medical provider for a treatment plan.

 Follow good hand-washing routines. Wash hands well and encourage your child to do the same.

 Make sure your child takes the prescribed medicine for the recommended time. This is important for the treatment to be effective.

Other caregivers should

 Tell parents if you notice a child has signs of ringworm.

 Notify parents to remove the child at the end of the program day and not return until treatment is started.

 Alert exposed staff and families to watch for signs.

 Observe children in the group when they arrive and during the day. Watch for any areas of skin or scalp that show signs of ringworm.

 Restructure dress-up play areas or any place where clothing or head-gear is shared. Make sure that equipment is laundered or sanitized between uses by different children.

 Avoid sharing dress-up articles or other clothing unless the fabric is washed between users or disposed of after one child uses it.

Child May Return to School or Child Care . . .

Once treatment is started.

Possible Cause: Roseola

What You Should Know

Roseola is a viral illness. It is mildly contagious. Signs of the disease are a skin rash and a high fever. It occurs in young children between 6 and 24 months old. The incubation period is from 9 to 10 days. One bout provides immunity.

What You Should Look For

- A persistent high fever (103° F or higher) lasting from 3 to 7 days
- Fever may cause seizure activity
- Often the child is not very ill when the fever is present
- Red, raised rash lasting from hours to several days that becomes apparent the day the fever breaks—usually the fourth day

What You Should Do

Parents or primary caregiver should

 Get medical care to make sure the disease is correctly identified.

 Get advice from your medical provider on what to do about the fever.

Other caregivers should

 Tell parents if you notice a child has signs of roseola.

Inform and reassure parents about the nature of the illness. Let them know that once the rash appears, the child is on the way to being well.

Child May Return to School or Child Care . . .

The child does not need to be kept from attending school or child care if his fever is not accompanied by a behavior change. The child may return when he feels well enough to do regular activities. If your child needs special care, the staff should decide if they can provide the care while still taking care of the other children in the group.

Possible Cause: Scabies

What You Should Know

Scabies is caused by mites that burrow under the top layer of the child's skin. The mites leave feces under the skin, which can cause intense itching. A medical provider may diagnose scabies by how the rash looks or by a skin scraping that shows a mite or egg. The mites are transferred by person-to-person contact. They are spread by sharing bedding, towels, or clothing. The child and all family members must be treated at home at the same time with prescription mite-killing cream or lotion. Itching can last from 2 to 4 weeks after treatment. The incubation period is from 4 to 6 weeks for people who have never had scabies before. The incubation period is from 1 to 4 days for those who have been infested before. Scabies affects people from all socioeconomic levels without regard to age or personal hygiene.

What You Should Look For

- Rash, severe itching (increased at night)
- Itchy red bumps or blisters found on skin folds between the fingers, toes, wrists, elbows, armpits, waistline, thighs, penis, abdomen, and lower buttocks
- Children younger than 2 years are likely to be infested on the head, neck, palms, and soles of feet; bumps or blisters may be scattered all over the body

What You Should Do

Parents or primary caregiver should

 Contact your medical provider for a treatment plan.

Follow package directions when applying the mite-killing lotion.

 Try to keep your child from scratching.

Treat all infected family members at the same time.

Machine wash all washable items in hot water. This includes bed linens, blankets, towels, clothing, jackets, and hats.

Use the hottest setting on the clothes dryer.

Place pillows and stuffed animals in a dryer on hottest setting for 30 minutes.

Leave items that cannot be washed or dried in a closed plastic bag for at least 4 days.

Other caregivers should

 Tell parents if you notice a child has signs and symptoms of the scabies.

 Alert exposed family members and staff to watch for signs.

Child May Return to School or Child Care . . .

After treatment is completed (treatment usually requires application of a lotion that stays on the skin overnight and then is washed off).

Possible Cause: Scarlet Fever (Scarlatina)

What You Should Know

Scarlatina is a bacterial infection that causes a generalized illness with a rash. The infection is from the same type of bacteria that cause strep throat. It is not more serious than strep throat. Scarlatina is contagious. It spreads from person to person by direct contact. A child also can get scarlatina by inhaling tiny droplets of infected secretions from the nose. Many people carry the strep bacteria in their nose and throat and are not sick. Illness caused by strep bacteria must be treated with an antibiotic. The incubation period is from 2 to 5 days.

What You Should Look For

- Rash appears mostly on trunk; it is most intense at under-arms, on groin, behind the knees, and on the inner thighs
- Rash is slightly raised fine bumps; the skin feels like fine sandpaper
- Painful sore throat in children older than 3 years of age; persistent nasal discharge and very bad smelling breath in children younger than 3 years of age
- High fever
- White coating on the tongue that changes to the appearance of a strawberry after 4 to 5 days
- Nausea, vomiting, and decreased appetite
- Swollen lymph nodes in the neck (swollen glands)
- Headache
- Skin peels after 1 week

What You Should Do

Parents or primary caregiver should

 Get medical care for diagnosis and treatment instructions.

 Follow instructions for treatment.

 Encourage child to drink clear fluids.

 Wash hands well after caring for child to reduce chance of spreading infection to yourself and others.

Other caregivers should

 Tell parents if you notice a child has signs and symptoms of scarlatina.

Alert parents whose children may have been exposed.

Child May Return to School or Child Care . . .

Twenty-four hours after antibiotic treatment has started. The child may return when he feels well enough to do regular activities. If your child needs special care, the staff should decide if they can provide the care while still taking care of the other children in the group.

Sore Throat

Possible Cause: Viral Sore Throat

What You Should Know

A viral sore throat is the most common cause of a sore throat. It is contagious. More than 90% of sore throats are viral. This type of sore throat will get better without treatment.

What You Should Look For

A throat that feels raw

What You Should Do

Parents or primary caregiver should

 Call your medical provider for a throat culture if symptoms last for more than 2 days.

 Encourage your child to drink fluids.

Wash hands well after caring for your child.

Do not allow your child to share toys that she puts in her mouth. Pacifiers, bottles, cups, or eating utensils also should not be shared.

Other caregivers should

 Tell parents if you notice a child has signs and symptoms of a sore throat.

 Do not allow children to share toys that they put in their mouths. Pacifiers, bottles, cups, or eating utensils also should not be shared.

If two or more children in the same group have the same symptoms, alert the families of the exposed children to watch for similar symptoms.

Child May Return to School or Child Care . . .

- Do not keep the child from attending school or child care unless she cannot swallow, is drooling a lot, is having breathing problems, or has fever with a behavior change.

- The child may return when she feels well enough to do regular activities. If your child needs special care, the staff should decide if they can provide the care while still taking care of the other children in the group.

Possible Cause: "Strep" Throat
What You Should Know

A strep throat is a bacterial infection caused by *streptococcal* bacteria. It occurs much less often than a viral throat infection. It is contagious. The bacteria are spread from person to person by direct contact. A child also can get scarlatina (scarlet fever) by inhaling tiny droplets of infected secretions from the nose. Many people carry the strep bacteria in their nose and throat and are not sick. When the strep bacteria take over as the most common germ in the tissue and cause illness, they must be treated with an antibiotic. A laboratory test is required to diagnose the infection with certainty. The incubation period is from 2 to 5 days.

What You Should Look For

Some of the following symptoms may be present:

* Sore throat
* Fever
* Stomachache
* Headache
* Swollen lymph nodes in neck
* Decreased appetite

Strep throat is much less likely if there is:

* Runny nose
* Cough
* Congestion

Children younger than 3 years rarely have a sore throat. It is more common for them to have persistent nasal discharge, sometimes with very bad smelling breath. They also may have fever, irritability, and loss of appetite.

What You Should Do
Parents or primary caregiver should

1. See your medical provider for diagnosis and treatment plan.

2. Make sure your child gets all of the prescribed antibiotic medicine. This will prevent relapse. Give all of the medicine even if the child seems to get better quickly.

Wash hands well after caring for your child.

 Do not allow your child to share toys that she puts in her mouth. Pacifiers, bottles, cups, or eating utensils also should not be shared.

Other caregivers should

 Tell parents if you notice a child has signs and symptoms of strep throat. Notify families of children who may have been exposed.

Child May Return to School or Child Care . . .

Twenty-four hours after antibiotic treatment has started. The child may return when she feels well enough to do regular activities. If your child needs special care, the staff should decide if they can provide the care while still taking care of the other children in the group.

Tooth Pain

Possible Cause: Bottlemouth Syndrome

What You Should Know

Bottlemouth syndrome is a special form of tooth decay in very young children. It is caused by prolonged exposure to milk or sugary liquids. Children at risk for bottlemouth syndrome take bottles of milk or juice to bed at naptime and bedtime. They also carry sugary beverages or milk around during the day. It is most common in the upper front teeth. Children with bottlemouth syndrome often need oral surgery with general anesthesia.

What You Should Look For

- Red gums
- Irritated mouth
- Teeth that do not look normal

What You Should Do

Parents or primary caregiver should

 Do not give your child a bottle of milk or juice (or any fluid containing sugar) at naptime, bedtime, or to carry around during the day. Only feed your child at specific meal and snack times.

Give your child water after a feeding to rinse sugary liquid off the teeth.

 Give only water or don't give a sleep-time bottle.

Other caregivers should

Talk with parents about the need to have the child's teeth examined by a medical provider.

Child May Return to School or Child Care . . .

The child need not be kept from attending school or child care.

Possible Cause: Cavities

What You Should Know

Cavities are caused by sticky foods that leave a sugar coating on teeth. This sugar feeds bacteria in the mouth. Then acid is produced that destroys the hard surface of the teeth. Some of the bacteria that do the most damage are transferred from the mouth of caregivers to children.

What You Should Look For

- Irritated mouth
- Sore gums
- Abnormal appearance of teeth
- Abnormal color of teeth

What You Should Do

Parents or primary caregiver should

 Avoid giving your child sticky foods between meals. These cling to teeth and cause decay. Some sticky foods are gummy, fruit-flavored treats, caramel candy, and licorice.

 Encourage your child to eat healthy snacks. Pretzels, raw vegetables, fresh fruit, and yogurt are good snack foods.

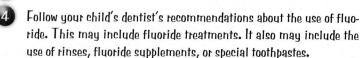 Encourage your child to brush or rinse teeth after snacks and meals.

Follow your child's dentist's recommendations about the use of fluoride. This may include fluoride treatments. It also may include the use of rinses, fluoride supplements, or special toothpastes.

Other caregivers should

Tell parents if you notice a child has cavities or other signs and symptoms.

Child May Return to School or Child Care . . .

The child need not be kept from attending school or child care.

Possible Cause: Teething

What You Should Know

Teething is gum pain caused by newly erupting teeth. It can be very painful. Teething can cause a child to be very cranky and have sleepless nights. It does not cause fever but can lead to an infection. This is because the child wants to put objects in his mouth.

What You Should Look For

- Crankiness
- Sleepless nights

What You Should Do

Parents or primary caregiver should

1. Provide teething toys for the child to chew.

2. Talk to your medical provider about using pain-reducing medicines, especially when the child is trying to sleep.

Other caregivers should

Tell parents if you notice a child has signs of teething.

Child May Return to School or Child Care . . .

The child need not be kept from attending school or child care. The child may return when he feels well enough to do regular activities. If your child needs special care, the staff should decide if they can provide the care while still taking care of the other children in the group.

Upper Respiratory Infection

Possible Cause: Common Cold

What You Should Know

An upper respiratory infection is a viral infection of the nose, throat, ears, and eyes. It is spread by direct or close contact with mouth and nose secretions. It is also spread by touching contaminated objects. The incubation period is from 2 to 14 days. The child is contagious a few days before signs or symptoms appear and while clear runny secretions are present.

What You Should Look For

- Cough
- Sore or scratchy throat or tonsillitis
- Runny nose
- Sneezing or nasal discharge
- Watery eyes
- Fever is low grade or does not exist
- Earache that may come after the secretions from a cold thicken; thick secretions can block the drainage tube that goes from inside the ear into the throat

What You Should Do

Parents or primary caregiver should

 Practice good hand-washing techniques.

 Teach your child to "give coughs and sneezes a cold shoulder." Use the shoulder or elbow to cover the nose and mouth when having to cough or sneeze if a tissue is not handy.

 Teach children to wash their hands after sneezing, coughing, or handling tissues.

 Dispose of tissues right away.

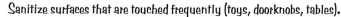 Sanitize surfaces that are touched frequently (toys, doorknobs, tables).

Ventilate rooms with fresh outdoor air.

Other caregivers should

Talk to parents about how to reduce the spread of cold viruses.

Child May Return to School or Child Care . . .

The child may return when he feels well enough to do regular activities. If your child needs special care, the staff should decide if they can provide the care while still taking care of the other children in the group.

Urination, Painful

Possible Cause: Urinary Tract Infection

What You Should Know

Most urinary tract infections are caused by bacteria. Urinary tract infections are more common in girls than boys. This is because girls have a shorter tube that connects the bladder to the outside (the urethra). Also, in girls, this tube is close to the anus. Bacteria in stool can easily get into the opening to the urinary tract. Boys do not usually get urinary tract infections unless they have some other health problem.

What You Should Look For

- Pain when urinating
- Increased frequency of urinating
- Fever
- Loss of potty training

What You Should Do

Parents or primary caregiver should

 Encourage children to drink enough fluids to keep their urine light yellow or clear like water. Very young children can learn that a dark urine color means they need to drink more.

 Teach girls to wipe only from front to back after toileting.

 Avoid using bubble bath products. They are a common cause of irritation of urinary and genital tissues. This makes it easier for a urinary infection to start, especially in girls.

 Get medical care promptly if you think your child has a urinary tract infection. The child will need to give a urine specimen for testing.

Follow your medical provider's instructions for treatment.

Other caregivers should

Alert the child's parents about any symptoms of urinary infection. Ask the parents to consult their medical provider.

Child May Return to School or Child Care . . .

The child may return when she feels well enough to do regular activities. If your child needs special care, the staff should decide if they can provide the care while still taking care of the other children in the group.

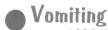 **Vomiting**

Possible Cause: Viral Gastrointestinal Infection

What You Should Know

Viral gastrointestinal infections often are contagious. They are less often caused by food poisoning or emotional upset.

What You Should Look For

* Diarrhea
* Vomiting
* Cramps

What You Should Do

Parents or primary caregiver should

 Manage vomiting by:
> ► Giving no food or fluid until 1 hour after vomiting has stopped.
> ► Giving clear fluids in small enough amounts so that no vomiting occurs. Start with an ounce of fluid. Then in 15 minutes, give half as much if that amount produces vomiting or twice as much in the next 15 minutes if that amount stays down.

 Consult your medical provider as soon as possible if:
> ► Vomiting continues, and the child has not urinated in 8 hours.
> ► Vomiting is associated with pain in the abdomen that doesn't go away.
> ► Vomit looks green or bloody.
> ► Child has had a recent head injury.
> ► Child looks or acts very sick.

Other caregivers should

 Remove child from the group if vomiting occurs more than once.

 Manage vomiting.

3 Inform parents that child vomited.

Child May Return to School or Child Care...

The child may return when he feels well enough to do regular activities. If your child needs special care, the staff should decide if they can provide the care while still taking care of the other children in the group.

Appendix B
First Aid Supply List

Here is a list of supplies that you might need when giving first aid care.

First Aid Supply List

Supply	Description
Adhesive bandages	These are a combination of a dressing and a bandage. They come in different sizes. Remember that plastic-backed bandages are a choking hazard. Use fabric-backed instead.
Adhesive tape or rolls of gauze	Use adhesive tape or rolls of gauze to hold a dressing in place over a wound.
Cold pack	Buy a reusable cold pack or use a plastic bag filled with ice. You can also use a bag of frozen vegetables. Be sure to wrap any type of cold pack in a thin cloth before putting it on a child's skin. Putting extreme cold directly on the skin can cause damage to the tissues.
Tissues, disposable	Use disposable tissues to avoid the spread of germs from cold or flu.
Towels, disposable	Use disposable towels, such as paper towels, for cleaning up spills of body fluids.
Elastic bandage	Put pressure on a bruised or swollen area by wrapping it in an elastic bandage.
Fever-reducing medicine	If your child has a fever and you have instructions from your medical provider, give a fever-reducing medicine. Examples of fever-reducing medicines are acetaminophen or ibuprofen. Do not give a child aspirin or products containing aspirin-like chemicals (salicylates).
Gauze pads	These can be used as a sterile dressing over a wound. They come in different sizes. Hold the gauze pad in place with adhesive tape or gauze from a roll.
Plastic-lined trashcan	Use a plastic-lined trashcan when cleaning up body fluids to dispose of contaminated items. Use another plastic-lined trashcan or pail to hold items that you will sanitize later.
Protective gloves	Use gloves that are nonporous, such as disposable medical gloves or rubber dishwashing gloves.

Sanitizing solution	You can buy a sanitizing solution or make your own. To make it, mix one-fourth cup of household bleach with 1 gallon of water, or 1 tablespoon of bleach to 1 quart of water. Leave this solution in contact with the surface for at least 2 minutes.
Soap	Any mild soap will work. Liquid soaps are better because they don't spread germs. Avoid soaps with heavy perfumes or those with abrasives. It is not necessary to use antibacterial soap.
Hand sanitizer	Use alcohol-based hand sanitizer when soap and water are not available to reduce the spread of germs.
Thermometer	A basic digital version may be the most practical and reliable way to determine if your child has a fever. (Do not use a mercury thermometer; the silver liquid inside is dangerous if the thermometer breaks.) Use a digital thermometer to take a rectal (in the bottom), oral (in the mouth), or axillary (under the arm) temperature. A tympanic (ear) thermometer, which is more expensive, is another option.
Tweezers	Use clean tweezers to remove splinters or other sources of puncture wounds and ticks that can be easily removed.

First Aid TIP

Don't use hydrogen peroxide for cleaning a wound. Wash the wound with soap and water. It is not necessary to put alcohol or antibiotic ointment on a wound unless your doctor tells you to.

First Aid TIP

Good hand washing is important to prevent the spread of many diseases. Here's the right way to wash your hands:

1. Use liquid soap, a disposable towel, and running water.
2. Wash your hands with soap and warm water for the amount of time that it takes to sing the "Happy Birthday" song twice.
3. Rinse your hands until they are free of soap and dirt.
4. Dry hands with a disposable towel or a single-use cloth towel.
5. If the faucet doesn't turn off by itself, use the towel to turn it off.

First Aid TIP

How to Take Your Baby's or Child's Temperature

Taking a rectal temperature:

▶ Clean the end of the thermometer with rubbing alcohol or soap and water; rinse in lukewarm water and dry. Apply a small amount of lubricant, such as petroleum jelly, on the end.

▶ Place your child tummy down across your lap. Hold the child by placing your palm against his lower back. Or, place the child face up and bend his legs to the chest. Rest your free hand against the back of the thighs.

▶ With the other hand, turn the thermometer on. Insert it to 1 inch into the anal opening (not too far). Hold the thermometer in place loosely with two fingers, keeping your hand cupped around your child's bottom. In about a minute, when you hear the beep, remove it and check the reading.

▶ Re-clean. Be sure the thermometer is labeled so it is not accidentally used in the mouth.

Taking an oral temperature:

▶ Wait 15 minutes after the child has been eating or drinking before taking a temperature.

▶ Clean the thermometer. Turn the thermometer on, and place the tip under the tongue toward the back of the child's mouth. Hold it in place for a minute until you hear a beep.

Taking an axillary temperature:

▶ Turn on the thermometer and place the small end in your child's armpit (thermometer should touch skin, not clothing).

▶ Gently hold the arm in place until the thermometer beeps.

Taking a tympanic temperature:

▶ The American Academy of Pediatrics advises against using this method for infants younger than 3 months. While a tympanic thermometer provides speedy results, the device needs to be inserted at the right angle in a child's ear to provide an accurate reading. Don't use these devices right after a child has been swimming or bathing or if ear pain is present.

▶ Place a clean cover on the cone-shaped end.

▶ Pull the ear backward slightly, and gently place the thermometer in the ear canal. Try to aim the probe toward the child's eye on the opposite side of the head.

▶ Turn on the thermometer; remove after it beeps.

Types of digital thermometers for use by age

Age	Technique/Type
Newborn to 3 months	Rectal (in the bottom)
3 months–3 years	Rectal, axillary (under arm), tympanic (ear)
4–5 years	Rectal, oral (in mouth), axillary, tympanic
5 years and older	Oral, axillary, tympanic

Source: AAP website. Wyckoff, A. S., "Thermometer Use 101." *AAP News*, vol. 30, no. 11, November 2009, p. 29.

GLOSSARY

A

abdominal thrusts A first aid technique used for a child who is choking to try to dislodge the foreign object from his airway.

absence seizures Seizures with a brief loss of responsiveness. The child will suddenly stare off into space for a few seconds and then become responsive again.

adhesive bandage Combination of a dressing and a bandage.

AED An automated external defibrillator is a small, electronic device that can analyze a heart rhythm and deliver a shock to help the heart start beating again. Use an AED for a victim in cardiac arrest as soon as one is available. Do not use an AED if a child is younger than 1 year old.

allergen A substance that causes an allergic reaction. Some common allergens are molds, dust, animal dander, pollen, foods, and medicines. Cleaning products and other chemicals are also common allergens. The body perceives allergens as dangerous.

allergic reaction The body's response to an allergen, often as hives or tissue swelling.

allergy An abnormal reaction of the body's immune system to a certain substance.

anaphylaxis A life-threatening type of allergic reaction that can cause the airway to swell.

antidote A substance that can counteract a poison.

arteries Large, deep, and well-protected blood vessels. Arteries carry blood away from the heart to all parts of the body. Large amounts of blood can be lost from arteries in a short amount of time. Bleeding from an artery may be life threatening.

aura A feeling that a grand mal seizure is about to begin.

B

back blows A first aid technique used for a baby who is choking to try to dislodge the foreign object from his airway; back blows are alternated with chest compressions.

bandage Holds the dressing in place. It also can be used to apply pressure to help control bleeding. Adhesive tape and rolls of gauze are often used as bandages.

blister A collection of fluid in a bubble underneath the skin.

body fluids All fluids that come from the body. These include urine, feces, saliva, blood, and vomit.

bruise Bleeding from blood vessels under the skin.

burn An injury to the skin that results from heat, chemical, electrical, or radiation damage to the body.

C

capillaries Tiny blood vessels located throughout the body. There are thousands of them. Bleeding is easy to control from capillaries.

carbon monoxide A deadly, invisible, odorless gas produced by equipment that burns fuel.

caregivers Legal guardians, relatives, and others who care for children.

chest compressions Pushing hard and fast on the chest of a person who is unresponsive and not breathing. Also, a first aid technique used for a baby who is choking to try to dislodge the foreign object from his airway; chest compressions are alternated with back blows.

closed fracture The skin is not broken at the location of the fracture.

concussion A brain injury that can range from mild to severe; some symptoms are headache, dizziness, nausea, confusion, drowsiness, or loss of responsiveness.

convulsive seizures Involuntary muscle contractions and body movement.

cornea The transparent outer covering of the eyeball.

CPR An abbreviation for cardiopulmonary resuscitation; CPR is emergency first aid for someone who is not responding and not breathing. To give CPR, the rescuer alternates compressing the chest to help keep blood circulating and giving rescue breaths to get air into the child's lungs. If available, an AED (automated external defibrillator) is used to help the heart start beating again.

crush injury An injury that results from squeezing or twisting a body part between two hard surfaces. Automobile accidents and hard falls can cause crush injuries.

cut An incision in the skin, which may be jagged or smooth. It may be shallow, like a paper cut, or deep. Cuts may be large or small.

D

deformity An abnormal shape caused by a broken bone.

dehydration A condition that results when the body doesn't have as much fluids as it needs. In hot weather this is caused by not drinking enough water to replace fluid that is lost through sweating.

diabetes A condition in which the body cannot regulate the sugars in the bloodstream.

direct pressure Pressing directly over a wound to stop bleeding, usually with a sterile dressing or clean, dry cloth.

dislocation The separation of a bone from a joint.

DOTS Memory aid for assessing bone, joint, and muscle injuries: Deformity, Open injury, Tenderness, Swelling.

224

dressing A clean covering placed over a wound. A gauze pad can be used as a dressing.

drooling Saliva that drips from a child's mouth. In healthy babies it is often a sign of teething. A child who is having trouble breathing may drool because of something in his throat that prevents him from swallowing. Another cause for drooling is that the child is making extra effort to breathe.

E

emergency medical services (EMS) A system of trained medical professionals who handle out-of-hospital emergencies. EMS is linked to a nationwide emergency phone number. In the United States, dial 911 to contact EMS.

epinephrine A hormone that stops the effects of anaphylaxis.

eye injury Injury to the eye, eyelid, and area around the eye.

eye trauma Any injury to the eye.

F

fainting A sudden and temporary loss of responsiveness caused by a brief lack of blood and oxygen to the brain.

febrile seizure A type of convulsive seizure that is caused by a rapid rise in body temperature.

first-degree burns Burns that involve only the top part of the skin.

flushing The skin on the child's face turns very red. Sometimes other areas of the body become red as well. Flushing can be a sign of a medical problem. Flushing is different from blushing. Blushing is usually a lighter pink or rose color. Blushing is associated with embarrassment.

fontanelle Opening in the skull of a young baby, often called a soft spot.

fracture A broken bone.

frostbite Tissue damage caused by extreme cold.

frostnip The most common local cold injury. Although ice crystals form, the tissue doesn't actually freeze. The ice crystals melt once the body part is warmed. With frostnip there is not much tissue damage.

G

generalized seizure with tonic-clonic movement A child who is having a grand mal seizure will become unresponsive for several seconds. Then he will have rhythmic stiffening and jerking of trunk and extremities.

Good Samaritan Law A law passed in many states to protect someone from legal liability when giving first aid in an emergency.

goose egg Swelling of the skin on the head that is shaped like a large egg.

grunting Noises that a child makes when trying to breathe better; may be a sign of trouble breathing.

gurgling Bubbling noises that you might hear in a child who is having trouble breathing.

H

head bobbing When a child's head bobs up and down with each breath; a serious sign that a child is having trouble breathing.

heat cramps Painful muscle spasms, usually in the legs and abdominal muscles. They are caused by dehydration.

heat exhaustion A condition that develops when children are exposed to hot temperatures for long periods of time. It often happens when they are actively playing and sweating. Heat exhaustion is caused by dehydration.

heat index The difference between the actual temperature and how hot it feels because of humidity and temperature.

heatstroke An illness that results when the body's natural cooling system does not work normally. The body is not able to make sweat as usual. This causes a dangerous rise in body temperature.

hyperglycemia Blood sugar levels in the body that are higher than normal.

hypoglycemia Blood sugar levels in the body that are lower than normal.

hypothermia A dangerous condition that can develop when children are exposed to cold temperatures for long periods of time. The temperature deep within the body drops below 95°F.

I

internal bleeding Bleeding in tissues far below the skin caused by an injury that is deep in the chest, abdomen, or brain.

internal head injury Damage to the brain. When the head receives a forceful blow, the brain strikes the inside of the skull. This causes some degree of injury.

L

ligaments The tissues that hold the joints together.

log roll A maneuver that helps to protect the neck and spine in case of injury.

M

mottling A blotchy "marble-like" look to the skin.

N

nematocysts Stinging tentacles fired by marine animals to capture their prey or to defend themselves.

nonconvulsive seizures Seizures with symptoms of confusion and loss of awareness.

nosebleed Bleeding from the nose caused by a broken blood vessel in the nostril.

O

open fracture There is an open wound over the fracture. The wound can be caused by the bone breaking through the skin. It also can be caused from the force that broke the bone.

open wound Broken skin as a result of an injury. Common types of open wounds are scrapes, cuts, broken blisters, punctures, and nosebleeds.

P

paralysis A loss of feeling and movement.

pediatric first aid The medical care that you give right away to a child who is injured or suddenly becomes very sick.

permanent teeth Teeth that develop at about 6 years old to replace primary teeth. By age 21 years, usually all 32 of the permanent teeth have erupted.

poison A substance that can cause harm to the body or even death if you eat, drink, touch, or breathe it.

Poison Help hotline A toll free number (1-800-222-1222) that you can call to find out what to do if your child gets a poisonous bite or sting. The advice is free and available 24 hours a day, 7 days a week, 365 days a year.

primary teeth Also known as baby teeth, primary teeth usually begin to grow at about 6 months old. Most children have a full set of primary teeth at about age 3.

protective gloves Nonporous gloves, such as disposable medical gloves or rubber dishwashing gloves.

puncture A small hole made in the skin, which may be deep or shallow. An example of a puncture wound is a splinter.

R

rabies A life-threatening viral disease in warm-blooded mammals that is most often transferred through bites.

rescue breathing A technique for getting air back into the lungs of a child who is not breathing.

RICE Memory aid for taking care of minor bone, joint, and muscle injuries: Rest, Ice, Compression, Elevation.

S

scrape An open wound that occurs when the top layer of skin is rubbed off. Because nerve endings just under the skin may be exposed, scrapes can be quite painful.

seal-like cough A barking "seal-like" cough may be a sign of croup and that the child is having trouble breathing.

second-degree burns Burns that blister and involve a deeper thickness of the skin.

seizures Medical conditions caused by a disturbance in the electrical impulses of the brain. Seizures can be either convulsive or nonconvulsive.

sniffing position A position a child may assume when having trouble breathing; the child will raise his head slightly and lean forward as if he is sniffing a flower.

snoring A rough or rattling sound with a low pitch that may be a sign that a child is having trouble breathing.

spinal cord The bony column that surrounds and protects the nerves of the spine.

spinal injury An injury that damages the spinal cord; moving a child with a spinal injury incorrectly may cause more damage. Spinal injuries are very serious and can result in paralysis and death. If you must move a child with a suspected spinal injury to keep him safe, use the shoulder drag method.

splinting Keeping an injured body part from moving.

sprain An injury to a ligament caused when the ligament is stretched beyond its limit.

strain An injury to a muscle caused when the muscle is stretched beyond its limit.

sunblock A barrier cream that prevents the UV light from reaching the skin.

sunscreen A chemical that bonds to the skin to prevent injury from UV light.

syrup of ipecac A medicine that causes vomiting; it is not recommended for use in a poisoning emergency.

T

tetanus A fatal disease caused when bacteria that live in the soil, in dust, and in human and animal feces enter the body through a wound. This disease causes strong spasms in the back, legs, arms, and jaw (lockjaw). Vaccinations protect against this disease.

third-degree burns The most serious types of burns that involve deeper tissues under the skin.

tripod position A position a child may assume when having trouble breathing; the child will lean forward with his arms straight. He usually props his hands on top of his knees.

U

universal distress signal The hands around the throat is the universal distress signal for choking.

V

veins Veins are located close to the surface of the skin. Veins can bleed heavily.

venom A poisonous fluid that insects and snakes make.

W

wheezing A whistling or squeaking sound that you hear when the child breathes out. This sound is caused by swelling or something blocking the small tubes in the lungs. Wheezing can come on suddenly. It can be a sign of an asthma attack.

wind chill The difference between the actual temperature and how cold it feels because of the wind.

INDEX

PHOTO CREDITS

Chapter 1
Opener © Corbis/age fotostock;
page 2 © Felix Mizioznikov/ShutterStock, Inc.

Chapter 2
Opener © SW Productions/Brand X Pictures/
Getty Images; page 15 © St. Bartholomew's
Hospital/Photo Researchers, Inc.

Chapter 3
Opener © Bubble Photolibrary/Alamy
Images; page 26-28 © Berta A. Daniels, 2010

Chapter 4
Opener © Stockbyte; page 34 © Gavel
of Sky/ShutterStock, Inc.; page 40 (top)
© Kiryay/ShutterStock, Inc.; (bottom)
© Katrina Brown/ShutterStock, Inc.;
page 47–48 © Berta A. Daniels, 2010

Chapter 5
Opener © DenisNata/ShutterStock, Inc.;
page 55 © Orange Line Media/ShutterStock,
Inc.; page 62 © Berta A. Daniels, 2010

Chapter 6
Opener © Andreas Wolf/age fotostock;
page 74 © Berta A. Daniels, 2010

Chapter 8
Opener © loriklaszlo/ShutterStock, Inc.;
page 85 © Rob Byron/ShutterStock, Inc.;
page 86 Courtesy of Dey, L.P.

Chapter 9
Opener © Daniel Prudek/ShutterStock, Inc.;
page 94 © Chuck Stewart, MD.; page 97
© Berta A. Daniels, 2010; page 98 (top)
© Alekcey/ShutterStock, Inc.; (middle)
© Kletr/ShutterStock, Inc.; (bottom)
© mathom/ShutterStock, Inc.; page 102
(left) © Joao Estevao A. Freitas (jefras)/
ShutterStock, Inc.; (right) © Petr Jilek/
ShutterStock, Inc.; page 103 Courtesy of
James Gathany/CDC; page 105 (top left)
© Photos.com; (top right) Courtesy of

Ray Rauch/U.S. Fish & Wildlife Service;
(bottom left) Courtesy of Luther C.
Goldman/U.S. Fish & Wildlife Service;
(bottom right) © SuperStock/Alamy Images;
page 106 (top) © photobar/ShutterStock,
Inc.; (bottom) Courtesy of Kenneth Cramer,
Monmouth College; page 108 © EcoPrint/
ShutterStock, Inc.

Chapter 10
Opener © Image Source/age fotostock;
page 112 © Berta A. Daniels, 2010; page 115
(top) © Thomas Photography LLC/Alamy
Images; (middle) © Thomas J. Peterson/Alamy
Images; (middle-bottom) Courtesy of U.S. Fish
& Wildlife Service; page 118 © Berta A. Daniels

Chapter 11
Opener © Apex News and Pictures Agency/
Alamy Images; page 121 © Dr. P. Marazzi/
Photo Researchers, Inc.; page 123 © Lonni
Aylett/Dreamstime.com; page 130 © Berta A.
Daniels, 2010

Chapter 12
Opener © Cordelia Molloy/Photo
Researchers, Inc.; page 139 Courtesy of Neil
Malcom Winkelmann

Chapter 13
Opener © Berta A. Daniels, 2010; page 147
© Berta A. Daniels, 2010

Chapter 14
Opener © Berta A. Daniels, 2010; page 155
© Berta A. Daniels, 2010

Chapter 15
Opener © Berta A. Daniels, 2010; page 157
© Renata Osinska/Fotolia.com

Unless otherwise indicated, all photographs
and illustrations are under copyright of
Jones & Bartlett Learning, courtesy of
Maryland Institute for Emergency Medical
Services Systems.